DR. NAGLER'S
BODY
MAINTENANCE
AND REPAIR BOOK

Willibald Nagler, M.D.
Irene von Estorff, M.D.

Illustrated by Nick Calabrese

SIMON AND SCHUSTER   New York

The information contained in this book is presented as a convenience to the reader. This book is not intended to replace the advice of a trained professional.

Designed by Irving Perkins Associates, Inc.
Manufactured in the United States of America
9 8 7 6 5 4 3 2 1

ACKNOWLEDGMENTS

We would like to thank James and Faith Stewart-Gordon, for their help in launching the project; A. E. Hotchner, for his thoughtful comments throughout the preparation of the manuscript; and Donald Hutter, for his sensitive editorial guidance.

—W. N.
—I.v.E.

CONTENTS

*Asterisks denote sections
with exercises.*

9

FOREWORD

A Western medical education today emphasizes two approaches to patient care: the surgical and the pharmacological—psychiatry also has its place. But there is a more recent and lesser-known fourth approach called physiatry, or physiatrics, or physical medicine and rehabilitation, and that is my specialty. The word physiatry derives from the Greek and denotes the treatment of disease processes by physical means, including exercise, heat, cold, prosthetics and orthotics, ultrasound, and electrical stimulation.

Our field is on the rise these days because our techniques are turning out to be effective for the entire musculoskeletal system—that is, for anything having to do with the muscles, ligaments, tendons, bones, joints, and nerves of the body. Which is not to say that surgery and medication have become any less valid, it is just that they have not provided some of the answers to certain medical problems that physical medicine has.

The field of physiatry is concerned not only with minor musculoskeletal injuries, but also with the unique problems of the severely disabled. The term "rehabilitation" has become part of medical nomenclature and is used to describe the specialized care that has evolved for such patients. It is also used in a more general sense to describe the *process* of recovery after an injury, through a structured treatment program based on the techniques of physical medicine. Thus, in 1947, the official name of our specialty became Physical Medicine and Rehabilitation, and the American Board of Physical Medicine and Rehabilitation was established to set training standards and requirements. To become a specialist in this field now requires four years of residency training and the passing of a set of rigorous written and oral examinations. There are currently 2,000 "physiatrists"—also known as physical medicine specialists or rehabilitation doctors—in the United States.

Perhaps a bit of background about myself and my practice will help you understand this field more clearly.

I was born in Austria and received my medical degree at the University of Vienna in 1958. Before starting what I thought would be a career as a country doctor back home, I came to the United States in order to broaden my clinical eperience and completed a residency program in Internal

Medicine at the Roswell Park Memorial Institute in Buffalo, New York, a well-known cancer center. I was also invited to work with my friend and colleague from Austria, Dr. Hans Kraus, who was practicing physiatry in New York City and, at the time, treating President John Kennedy's back ailment. Dr. Kraus needed a "backup" in case he could not be available on short notice for the president, and so I came to New York to fill this role and to pursue my interest in rehabilitation medicine. Eventually, I decided to settle in this country and devote myself to this area of specialization. Today I am professor and head of the Department of Rehabilitation Medicine at The New York Hospital–Cornell Medical Center, and I am also chief of the Rehabilitation Service at Memorial Sloan-Kettering Cancer Center. During the last two decades, I have been involved in treating a wide variety of musculoskeletal problems in patients of all ages, from everyday back, shoulder, and neck ailments to the more severe and disabling effects of cancer, stroke, congenital defects, spinal cord injury, amputation, and burns. I am fortunate to have a dedicated staff of six physiatrists besides myself, eight residents-in-training and sixty-five physical and occupational therapists involved in caring for the patients we see at both hospitals.

When I first came to this country, I had considerable difficulty making myself understood in English. A college professor, whom I was caring for as a patient, suggested that I obtain a book for younger readers and read it out loud, concentrating on the pronunciation and intonation of each syllable and word. I chose a textbook on American history and carried it as often as possible to the roof of the hospital where I was training and practiced reading aloud. One afternoon I happened to be reading from the Declaration of Independence when one of the hospital employees opened the door to the roof. He heard my voice, listened to the words I was spouting, and called the police. He thought I was a dangerous radical, possibly even a revolutionary, plotting the overthrow of the government! When the police arrived and I explained what was going on, they were very amused. But the incident could have been avoided if I had had a chance to explain to the hospital worker what I was doing and clear up his hasty misinterpretation of my actions.

I always think of this incident as a prime example of the importance of communicating with those around you. In all areas of medicine, mutual understanding and clear lines of communication are vitally important. An internist has to be able to explain to you why he is prescribing a certain medication and what its side effects may be; you, in turn, are responsible for taking the medication according to a certain schedule, and for reporting to your internist how you are responding to it. Or, a surgeon needs to explain why he is operating, what the risks are, and what he hopes to achieve; you will be required to follow his instructions for medication and physical activity in the post-operative period, and to keep him informed on how you are feeling. In both cases, you are a partner in the management of your own health.

What makes the field of physical medicine and rehabilitation a little different is that you are an *active* member of this partnership. For example, what you tell me about how you feel is especially important in helping me make the right diagnosis because laboratory tests are seldom useful in this field and I can't do an exploratory operation on you. Even X-rays and CAT (computerized axial tomography) scans can not always give you all the answers. And when it comes to treatment, you are truly active, performing the exercises that have been shown to you, finding a way to integrate them into your daily schedule. This is a lot more demanding than taking a pill three times a day with meals! To monitor your progress, I also need a lot of feedback from you because, again, there is no simple test to help me. I have to rely heavily on what you say and how you look and act. I have to examine you carefully each time I see you. I also have to be absolutely clear about what I find on my examination, what I want you to do, what adjustments have to be made as we go along. I know that if I explain the anatomic and physiologic principles behind the exercise program I am prescribing, you will be more likely to carry it out. But I still have to count on you to take the initiative in following through on my instructions and in keeping me posted on your progress.

To write a single book about the broad spectrum of patients that are included in a physiatrist's practice would be, in my opinion, an impossible undertaking. What I do here is share with you what I have learned over the years about the most common musculoskeletal problems that afflict large segments of the population; how I, as a physiatrist, approach these problems; and how you, as the patient or potential patient, can become a partner in the prevention and management of such problems.

In my work I am like a detective of the body, working with the clues that you give me with your story, that I observe, and that I feel with my hands. Isaac Stern, the famous violinist, came to us because he had developed a cramping in his fingers without having made any conscious change in his technique. I couldn't figure out what was wrong at first, so I asked him to return with his violin, which he did. Over and over he played portions of Bach's Brandenburg concertos, until I saw what was wrong. With a properly designed exercise program and the willingness to carry it out, he was able to overcome the problem and return to his usual superb playing form.

In the context of modern medicine, our ideas may seem "new," but in actuality they stem from centuries of clinical experience with, and interest in, the muscles of the body, fitness, and exercise. Ancient medical writings from India and Greece make frequent references to therapeutic exercise and massage. We know that Hippocrates advocated exercise for the treatment of certain injuries, and that the Greek physician-anatomist Galen acted as a physical therapist to the gladiators in Rome. Wherever there have been athletes preparing for competition, or soldiers for battle, there has been interest in fitness and training and the repair of injury.

What *is* new is modern medicine's growing recognition of the inadequacy or inapplicability of some of its traditional approaches and techniques for the diagnosis and treatment of many musculoskel-etal problems. The importance of exercise and other physical measures is being redis-covered, so to speak. Also new is the up-surge of interest in our area of medicine on the part of the general population. Why now? In large part I believe it's because of the unprecedented switch from passive ob-server to participant in athletic activity and exercise that has occurred in this country. Why this phenomenon should be taking place just at this time is for the sociologists to determine, but apparently there has never been anything quite like it in West-ern history. Millions of people are running, exercising, and participating in sports on a regular basis. And they are doing it, or starting it, at a later period of life than ever before. The medical field has had to re-spond to these developments, and in doing so, it has been learning a great deal about the use of physical means to benefit human health.

It is ironical, then, that this boom in physical activity has, in turn, focused at-tention on our sedentary life-styles, which until recently we assumed were protecting us from musculoskeletal injury. While all sorts of machines and gadgets spare us from overexertion, we are still, for too much of our daily lives, sitting at our desks and allowing our abdominal muscles to become slack, our back muscles to tighten up, and our posture to deteriorate. The next thing we know, we have back prob-lems—today more than ever a major ail-ment in this country. And we wonder why! Enter physical medicine. Analysis of the biomechanical structure of the back and its component parts—one of the fundamen-tals of physical medicine—helps us under-

stand how a back injury occurs, and what we can do about it.

There is another set of problems, a dif-ferent risk for people who have made, or are planning to make, the rather sudden transition to a more active life-style. Unless they are gradually trained within the framework of a structured, individualized program under the guidance of a knowl-edgeable professional, muscles that are out of shape can be injured quite easily *during* exercise. Unfortunately, too many health clubs and exercise books encourage you to plunge right into relatively vigorous rou-tines before your muscles are ready. Mus-cle tears or other injuries can then, all too easily, discourage you from following through on your good intentions.

Along with all of this upsurge of interest and participation in exercise and athletic activities has come a great deal of curiosity about the body. Is exercise really good for you? If it is, how can you keep yourself as fit as possible? What can you do to prevent injury? Is there anything you can do on your own to help repair an injury? When should you go to a doctor?

These are the issues this book addresses, and the questions it tries to answer. It fo-cuses on exercise as both a therapeutic dis-cipline and a form of preventive medicine. It offers you a broad education in physiat-ric medicine and the musculoskeletal workings of your body. And it teaches you some important principles of body mainte-nance and repair.

Our book is divided into two parts. In the first and shorter section, we offer a gen-eral understanding of good (and not so good) exercise mechanics leading into a basic program that, if conscientiously followed, can serve as your lifetime foundation for sound physical fitness. The second and main part of the book contains a comprehensive, alphabetic guide, an encyclopedia to use as your personal reference to the various components of the body, what can go wrong with them, and physiatric resources for their repair, with specific exercise programs and detailed therapeutic instructions.

Like any delicate machine, the body must be looked after. The potential for injury can never be completely eliminated because the body is constantly being subjected to unexpected stresses and strains. But good maintenance will cut down significantly on the frequency of injury. And you will be surprised by how much *you* can do to help repair the body when injury does occur.

PART ONE

FITNESS THROUGH EXERCISE:
Your Foundation for Body Maintenance

The Case for Exercise

To prove something beyond the shadow of a doubt in medicine is always difficult because so many overlapping factors are involved. Nevertheless, it is safe to say that the benefits of exercise for general well-being have been shown to far outweigh the risks. Not all patients with pneumonia will die if they don't receive antibiotics, but no one today would take a chance and withhold them. I feel the same way about a sedentary life-style and exercise: I couldn't advise an individual to continue such a life-style when I know that exercise can help build defenses against disease and injury. We still have much to learn about a specific "dosage" for a given individual, but the overall benefits cannot be denied.

Still, many people remain frightened of exercise. If someone dies of a heart attack at home, it is likely to be mentioned on the obituary page; but if someone dies while jogging in the park, it becomes a news item. Yet even this type of publicity can have a positive effect as it leads more and more people to undergo cardiovascular testing before they start on a new exercise regimen. Anyone over thirty-five can tell from such "stress" testing—which should be done in conjunction with a blood analysis of one's cholesterol count and triglyceride levels—whether an underlying condition exists that would preclude a vigorous regimen.

Most beneficial to the body's cardiovascular health is aerobic exercise: sustained activity that makes maximum use of the body's oxygen. Any kind of exercise that makes the heart and lungs work harder to provide an adequate oxygen supply to the muscles is by definition aerobic. Brisk walking, running, swimming, and bicycling are all excellent aerobic exercises. For maximum benefit, such sustained vigorous activity for twenty minutes at a time, three days a week, is generally recommended for good physical maintenance. The resultant increased capacity of the heart to pump blood and the lungs to exchange oxygen reduces the ill effects of coronary disease. A well-trained heart-lung system will, therefore, also help someone *with* heart disease to live much better—and maybe even longer.

Anaerobic exercise—activity too brief to make use of the body's oxygen—does not appear to provide any long-term benefit to the cardiovascular system, although it can build up muscles. Anaerobic exercise comes in short bursts, usually less than a minute. The energy for such physical surges derives not from oxygen drawn into the lungs but from the substance glycogen, a carbohydrate that is stored in the muscles themselves. This short-term supply is always ready for instant use, but it is only adequate for highly intense activity. The 100-yard dash, one of the most demanding of all competitive endeavors, is an example of an anaerobic event. It doesn't last long

21

enough to be anything else! Many sports that appear to epitomize fitness are really more anaerobic than aerobic. Football and baseball require more anaerobic energy than aerobic capacity—participation consists of short bursts of action followed by longer periods of relative inactivity.

Building up your cardiovascular system through regular, sustained periods of aerobic exercise should be paralleled by improving the flexibility and strength of your musculoskeletal system. If your muscles and joints can't keep up with your jogging or bicycling, you may develop some minor injuries that will slow you down or even force you to give up exercising altogether. I frequently see examples of this dilemma at New York Hospital.

The important thing to realize is that our aerobic capacity is one of the most precious physical resources we have, that it can be significantly improved with a small amount of effort, and that the muscles and joints should be given equal attention so that the rest of the body can keep up with the heart and lungs.

Risky Exercise and Fitness Fads

Our perception of the value of certain individual exercises has changed in the last decade—to a large degree in the relatively new light of physiatry—and thus some traditional exercises are now considered undesirable and, in some cases, even risky.

The straight-leg sit up is a good example. Once considered the most fundamental of exercises, this form of sit-up, with the legs out straight and held by a partner, can put excessive strain on low back muscles and ligaments, and it doesn't really do what it's supposed to do: strengthen the abdominals. There are a number of variations for this basic exercise, but the right way to do a sit-up is to bend your knees and curl up with your shoulders.

Deep knee bends, another traditional exercise, can be dangerous if you go all the way down and actually touch your buttocks to your heels. Why? Because you are overworking your knee joints, and thereby risking ligament and cartilage damage. If you wish to do deep knee bends (they are a good strengthener for the quadriceps muscle), do them so that at their lowest point your thighs are parallel to the ground.

Toe touching with legs straight, especially when you bounce to try to close the gap, is another exercise to be avoided because it can strain the lower back. So can lifting heavy weights over your head the way strongmen do in the circus. Working out with weights that are smaller and lighter, however, can be an effective means of building up muscle strength.

Another problem area is your neck, with its complex network of nerves and blood vessels. Any exercise or treatment that tips the head back very forcefully can have dangerous consequences. I have seen cases involving yoga positions, gymnastic maneuvers, and push-ups with the legs raised above head level in which the blood supply to the spinal cord was actually cut off and produced permanent damage. Just looking up at the ceiling can be a problem for older individuals when bony osteoarthritic changes narrow the vertebral openings through which arteries pass. (That's why older people should be extremely careful about working on ladders or standing on stools, performing any type of task—such as changing light bulbs—that tips the head back. Such a position can reduce blood flow to the spine and brain for an instant, which is long enough to cause a blackout and fall.)

A lot of my new patients come to me expecting shortcuts to health. There are no shortcuts. Unfortunately, that doesn't stop people from trying to find them! There are probably more fitness fads and gimmicks on the market today than ever before. Not all such programs and devices are necessarily harmful or potentially dangerous, it's just that they may keep you from doing what's really best for you, without your realizing it.

No matter how good our intentions, or perhaps *because* of them, most of us can be highly susceptible to claims of health benefits, or at least what may appear to be beneficial to our health at a particular time or place. Let me give you an example. When I was a boy in Austria, I had a difficult and debilitating case of asthma. As a result, a number of doctors came to our house to examine me and offer cures. They finally concluded that the very best thing for me to do was to drink raw milk, just as it emerged from the cow. At that time this was thought to be healthful and beneficial. My grandmother was all for it, too, and so I drank glass after glass of raw milk. I choked down every glass, yet it did nothing to help my asthma. But something did seem to be happening to the cow! The poor animal got thinner and thinner, and finally became so emaciated that it had to be sold to the local butcher. I thought it was my fault, but when this fine gentleman slaughtered my milk cow, he found it riddled with tuberculosis! Fortunately, the milk didn't hurt me—indeed, I probably built up a tremendous immunity to the kind of TB cows get! But I was lucky.

Such is the extent of the fitness boom that all of us, at one time or another, may be tempted to take a sip of raw milk because it's easy or popular. My advice: Beware of anything that makes excessive claims and unrealistic promises, whether it involves diet, health, or fitness. Almost certainly, the main benefits will be to the financial well-being of the manufacturer.

Gravity boots, those expensive contraptions that include attachments for your feet and a metal frame from which you hang upside down, are a good example of the raw milk of the fitness boom. The idea, I guess, is to sort of stretch out and straighten your spine, thereby relieving it of tension and pain. Aside from the fact that the spine cannot be straightened even by accepted methods of traction, I fail to see any benefit whatsoever from such equipment, unless you're interested in hanging head down and doing sit-ups in the air, a possible way to build strong stomach muscles. A patient of mine once bought me a pair of gravity boots, not because of my back, which is fine, but because she had read that they can make you *taller,* and while apparently she found me personable enough, she thought my height could use some modification. While I do appreciate her concern, I will wait until more studies have been done on gravity boots. Meanwhile, I don't advise using the equipment, especially if you're thirty-five years of age or older, because it can send your blood pressure soaring. And if you have glaucoma or hypertension (and, most especially, if you don't know it) such rapid shifts in blood pressure can be extremely dangerous.

Running with weights wrapped around your ankles has some virtues, for it makes your body lift more pounds and thus work harder. But this particular glass of raw milk has been oversold, in my opinion, and certainly I would not recommend it for anyone in their fifties or sixties. Running with ankle weights makes it all too easy to pull a muscle—in the groin area, for example—which can be painful and disabling, to the point of keeping you from doing any exercise for several weeks.

The rubber suits that some people wear while working out—supposedly to lose weight—can also be dangerous to your health. When you exercise, your body generates heat and works hard to dispose of it in a variety of ways, including the release of perspiration. Rubber suits hold heat and perspiration against your skin and make it more difficult for your body to get rid of them, which in turn makes your heart work harder. Such suits are useless except for skin diving.

Aerobic dancing may be appropriate if you don't like to exercise alone and are willing to pay in order to increase your heart rate. But you can accomplish exactly the same thing by walking briskly, jogging, or running. And I'm especially concerned about aerobic dancing for older people and those who are overweight. Classes are often conducted in warm, poorly ventilated rooms, and if you are older or overweight, you may be subjecting yourself to considerable risk. You may injure your joints and muscles or upset your cardiovascular system.

It can also be risky to follow exercise programs on television or off videotapes. Some of these programs move so quickly that you really can't keep up with them. And if you try without having warmed up adequately beforehand, you can hurt yourself. I see and treat such injuries all the time.

The variety of "muscle-toning" machines that have sprung up in the last decade, first in college and professional gyms and now on the home front, is staggering. The Nautilus machine, for example, is well-designed and effective in its capacity to exercise opposing muscle groups sequentially. The principle is a good one: You use one set of muscles moving out or up, then a second group on the way back. A constant resistance is applied in both directions throughout the range of motion. But I can rig up something similar at home, working with pulleys and ropes and weights, and it's a lot cheaper.

Home workout machines are now widely and heavily advertised. If you are interested in one, I would urge you to confer with a physiatrist or some other well-qualified doctor before you spend your money. Resistance exercise using maximum weights raises blood pressure, without aerobic benefit, and tight muscles can tear when subjected to enthusiastic but untutored stressing. (For more on home exercise equipment, see page 100.)

So, you should look into new products and programs very, very carefully. Be sure you understand just what the purpose of the exercise is, and try to establish credible medical evidence for the usefulness and safety of any device. The next time you hear of an attractive new program or gadget, ask yourself: Is this a glass of raw milk?

As We Get Older

During the last decade I have seen more older people making good use of their natural physical resources than ever before. I remember when male patients in their fifties and sixties would arrive at my office complaining of aches and pains from head to toe. They were usually overweight, had difficulty moving about, and many of them smoked heavily. Today, they are much slimmer, more active, and more likely to be nonsmokers. Instead of needing treatment for severe aches and pains, they now come for advice on how to train their muscles for a more effective overhead smash on the tennis court, or how to cut down on feelings of soreness after running for several miles!

The leader of a Mt. Everest–bound expedition may be a man in his sixties; the winner of a solo sailing race across the Atlantic may be no younger. Many of our astronauts are superbly fit, active men in their fifties. They have learned to overcome what used to be considered the inevitable by-products of aging: creaky joints, body stiffness, soreness, and quick fatigue. Yet still too many of us are afflicted with a kind of "body rust" produced by chronic inactivity and lack of exercise. And while it is true that aging *does* produce changes in the musculoskeletal system, much can now be done to counteract these changes.

In 1970, there were 20 million people sixty-five years of age or older in this country; by 1990, there will be 10 million more, including 3 million over the age of eighty-five. So it has become all the more important to understand what happens as we get older.

One of the first noticeable signs of aging is a change in the quality of a person's motion. One can't reach as far as one used to, and quick, sudden movements don't come as easily. No doubt we lose a certain percentage of joint mobility as a result of the tightening of the capsule in the joint, which is caused by aging, but most of the range of motion we lose as we get older is attributable to a sedentary, convenience-oriented way of life that takes all the impetus out of performing those activities which require physical skill and range of motion. We are surrounded by so-called work-saving devices of all kinds.

It is well-established that most of us lose about 30 percent of our original hip mobility by age forty. While this still leaves sufficient range to play, say, tennis, we will continue to stiffen up as the years go by *unless* we exercise properly. It has been found that gymnasts who keep exercising can maintain their full range of motion for many many years. Other studies have shown that older persons who participate in a twelve-week aerobic training program noticeably increase the range of motion in their joints. So not all changes from aging are inevitable; they can respond to individually maintained exercise.

Besides joint stiffness, there is also some selective weakening and shortening of the muscles with aging. Again, I am quite sure this is mostly caused by our way of life rather than by intrinsic factors. Shortening is particularly prevalent in the pectoralis muscles of the chest, in the thigh or hip flexor muscles, and in the hamstring muscles at the back of the legs—all of them muscles that tend to weaken from disuse. Furthermore, there is a weakening of the scapular adductor muscles—the muscles that pull the shoulder blades together and help keep the upper back straight—contributing to a stooped posture. To be sure, there is a selective weakening of the stomach muscles that is at least partly caused by skeletal changes—that is, the distance between the rib cage and pelvis becomes a bit shorter as we grow older because the disks in our spine dry out and become thinner—and the bony parts of the spine may themselves become weakened and lose some of their height, resulting in further slackening of the stomach muscles. Still, much of the aggregate effect of this problem also comes from inactivity.

You may well ask whether stiff joints or tight and weak muscles really make any difference to your health and well-being. Of course they do. If the range of motion in your joints is well-maintained, you will be able to continue participating in exercise and athletic activities for many years to come, and with reduced risk of injury. Furthermore, you will in turn be more likely to maintain aerobic levels of exercise in those kinds of activities that help make your bones stronger. If you look at pictures of your not so distant ancestors, you will see that most of them became stooped in old age with their neck and head bent forward. This was a result of osteoporosis, which weakens bony structures and causes changes in the configuration of the vertebral column. Now that we know much more about our nutritional and calcium needs, and the positive effect of certain kinds of exercise on our bony metabolism, we are already seeing less and less of this condition. Changes in our skeletal structure can't be totally prevented, but we can do a lot to mitigate them as we get older.

The main thing to remember is that while there are a variety of reasons for "stiffening up" with age, the most important seems to be simple inactivity. With a well-outlined exercise program, many of these changes can be overcome. It's never too late: you can start at any age. But first, you should check out your condition for any such program.

The Nagler Test

A sustained exercise program makes demands of certain parts and systems of the body, and it is wise to know beforehand how your body measures up, and to correct any potential problems before they can become aggravated in a regimen. As previously mentioned, it is a good idea to undergo a stress test before starting an aerobic program, especially for the first time, but that won't tell you anything about your musculoskeletal condition. And you can't do a stress test yourself. I have therefore devised a simple, seven-part test to evaluate not only your aerobic capacity, but also the flexibility of certain muscle groups and the strength of your abdominal muscles. This test can be taken safely by anyone at any age, whether you are completely out of shape or are already involved in some form of exercise and athletics. You may *seem* altogether fit and still have poor endurance, or tight muscles prone to injury, or weak abdominals with a potential for causing problems in the back. These exercises will gauge your readiness to undertake an aerobic regimen, and they suggest remedial exercises for any basic deficiencies.

TEST 1

Walk for 20 minutes outdoors, then, with hands behind your back, climb a flight of stairs that has at least 20 steps. If you are out of breath when you reach the top and your quadriceps (the large muscle in front of the thigh) feel a strain, or your knees feel wobbly, you are in poor aerobic condition. No special corrective exercise is indicated, but clearly you *need* the aerobic program that begins in the next section.

TEST 1

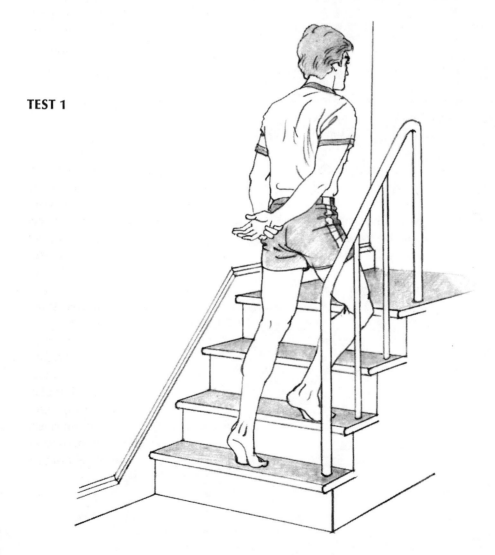

TEST 2

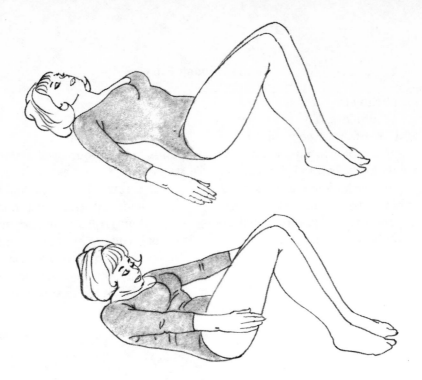

TEST 2

This is a test of your abdominal muscle strength. Lie on your back with your knees bent and slightly apart from each other, feet flat on the floor, and arms extended alongside your hips. Curl your head and shoulders forward until you are in a half-sitting position and hold for five seconds (see illustration). Do as many sit-ups as you can. You should be able to do 20 to 25 without difficulty. If you can't, start exercising your abdominal muscles (see the exercises included in "Stomach Muscles," starting on page 250).

TEST 3

This is a test for hip flexor stiffness. Lie on your back on a firm surface. Bend one leg to the chest and grasp firmly around the lower leg; press the back of the knee of the other leg down onto the surface while stretching your heel forward. If you feel pain or tightness in the groin area of the straight leg, it is time for you to do some hip stretching exercises (see pages 144 and 153, exercises 5 and 18).

TEST 3

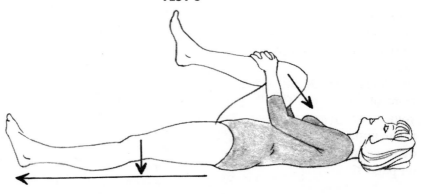

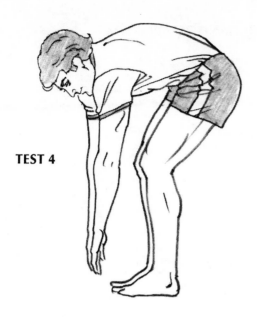

TEST 4

TEST 4

This is a test for tightness of your hamstring muscles in the back of the thigh, and your back extensor muscles located along the spine, from the neck to the waist. From the waist, with your arms hanging loosely and knees bent slightly, bend forward and try to touch your toes. Exhale as you bend forward. If you cannot come close to your toes, and you feel tightness in the lower back or in your hamstrings, you definitely need stretching exercises for your back extensor muscles and hamstrings (see exercises 4 and 8 on pages 43 and 47).

TEST 5

This exercise tests the tightness of your shoulder and upper back muscles. Sit in a straight-backed chair with your feet flat on the floor. Place your hands on top of your shoulders. Try to touch your elbows in front of your chest, exhaling as you bring your elbows together. If you feel tightness in the upper back or shoulders, it is time to do some stretching exercises (see exercise 3 on page 42).

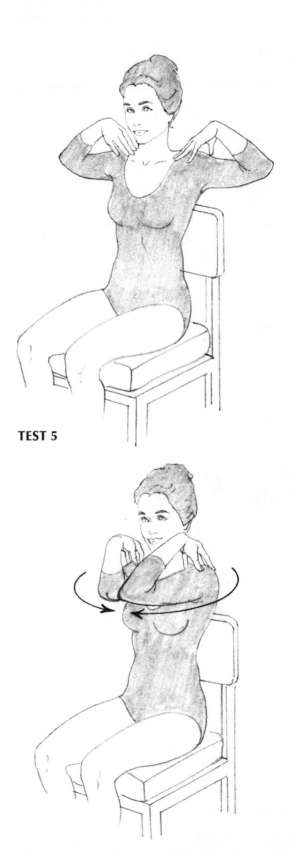

TEST 5

TEST 6

This exercise is a test for tightness of your calf muscles, or, as they are often called, heel cords. Stand 11 inches from a wall. Place the palms of your hands on the wall at shoulder height. Step back with your right foot an additional 11 inches, placing your heel flat on the floor. Keeping your right heel on the floor and the knee tight, lean toward the wall by bending your arms at the elbows and your left knee slightly. If you feel a substantial pull on the calf of the right leg, you have tight heel cords and it is time for stretching (see exercise 10 on page 49). Check your left heel cord in the same manner.

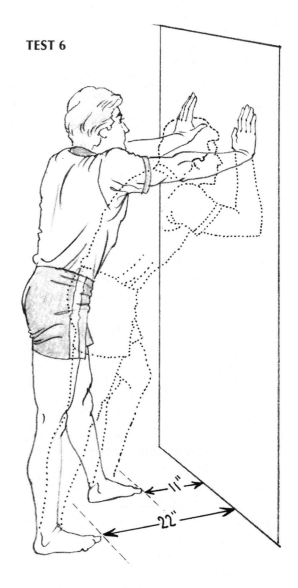

TEST 6

TEST 7

This is a test for tightness of your hamstrings alone. Lie on your back, knees bent, hands and arms at your sides, and feet flat on the floor. Bring the right knee to your chest, then straighten the knee and flex your foot so that the toes point toward the knee. If you feel tightness in your hamstrings while the leg is at about a 60-degree angle, it is time for hamstring stretching.

TEST 7

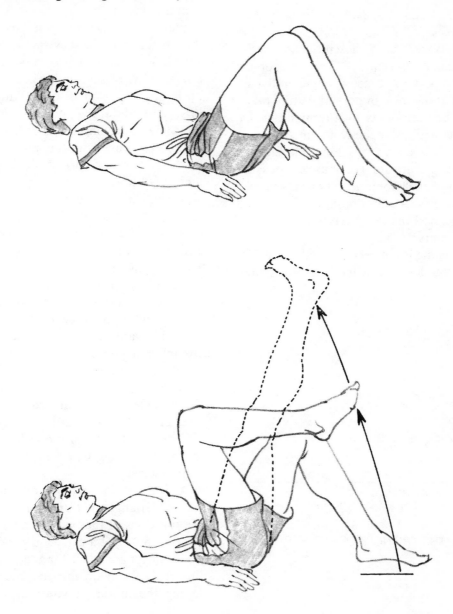

The Triangle of Fitness Program

For a full and clear perspective on the effectiveness of regular exercise for body maintenance, I have chosen the concept of a "Triangle of Fitness." The base of the triangle is aerobic activity, generally accepted as the most important feature of exercise because of its long-term protective benefits and its capacity to fine-tune the body as a heart-lung machine. The sides of the triangle are for the muscles, because without them aerobic activity is impossible. The better shape they're in, the better you will feel and the less likely you will be to injure yourself.

Stretching is represented on the left side. Most muscles have a tendency to tighten up when not used regularly. If suddenly stretched—as when you lunge for a volley on the tennis court, or even do something as simple as reach for the phone—they can go into spasm: very strong, tight, and painful contractions of the muscle fibers that continue involuntarily.

Warm-ups also belong on the left side of the triangle because they should always be a prelude to stretching or any other exercise activity. Most people choose to warm up by jogging in place or walking around briskly for about five minutes. Or you can do some mild limbering exercises—very relaxed movements of the muscles without holding them on stretch—for the same amount of time.

Strengthening is represented on the right side of the triangle. This keeps the mechanical units of the body properly aligned and helps improve the oxygen-delivery system to the muscles.

Generally speaking, progress through a full exercise program proceeds clockwise around the triangle, beginning on the left side with warm-up and stretching, through strengthening on the right, to aerobic activity along the base.

Cool-downs also belong on the base of the triangle as the final phase of all exercise. They allow the cardiovascular system and its distribution of blood flow through the body to readjust gradually to a lower activity level.

Another useful analogy, one that parallels the Triangle of Fitness, is to compare the functions of the body through exercise to the running of a car. Doing such warm-ups as jogging in place for a few minutes or limbering the main muscle groups is like letting the motor of your car run for a

STRETCHING
(Preceded by Warm-Up)

STRENGTHENING

AEROBIC ACTIVITY
(Followed by Cool-Down)

THE TRIANGLE OF FITNESS

while on a cold morning. The heart and engine are primed for action as blood and fuel travel through their respective circuits. The temperature of the component parts is raised and renders them less susceptible to injury or damage.

Stretching of the muscles may be seen as a form of lubrication. By lessening the pull of muscles at their attachment sites, there is less friction as they move over joints and bones, and therefore less chance of wear and tear. Strengthening is analagous to tune-ups, particularly measures that secure the various body parts neatly in place so they can work together efficiently. Loose or unstable parts in any system have the potential for causing injury and damage. The effect of aerobic exercise can be compared to the boost of a fuel injection system. It enables you to make optimal use of the energy supply available.

No man-made machine, however, can equal the complexity and versatility of the body. For the body, as a living organism, is capable of changing, improving, and repairing itself. It may be more difficult to predict or control its condition on a minute-to-minute basis, but it can be maintained by understanding how to use exercise as a foundation for fitness and prevention of injury. And that is the aim of our Triangle of Fitness program.

If you are not already engaged in a sport or some regular exercise activity, the best way to approach any fitness routine is to *ease into it* at whatever pace is most comfortable for you, and not get too caught up in a rigid schedule that allows for no flexibility on a day-to-day basis. A lot will depend on your age. If you are older and have been out of shape for many years, you

should take much longer than a younger person to proceed around the triangle. (And you shouldn't feel bad about it!) Too many fitness books on the market are geared toward people in their twenties, and it can be quite discouraging if you are older and feel you just can't keep up with the pace.

For purposes of an overall norm, I like to think in terms of a six-week period for each of the three components of the program: stretching, strengthening, and aerobic activity. As a clinical observation not based on any scientific studies, I find this to be a rather natural cycle for the muscles. If you are in your twenties, you could cut each or any of the periods down to two to three weeks; if you are in your sixties, you could extend it to two to three months.

The program can proceed in either of two ways. One can move around the triangle sequentially: first, a period of stretching exercises conducted every day; second, a period of strengthening exercises conducted five or six times a week at the beginning, then three times a week, with stretching exercises continuing daily; and third, a period of aerobic activity—at least twenty minutes at a time, three times a week—with daily stretching and strengthening exercises at least three times a week. Or, you may wish to save time by starting the stretching program and aerobic activity at a milder level simultaneously, gradually working in the strengthening program (the only leg of the triangle that requires a preparatory period, whether of stretching alone or stretching and aerobics).

At the end of this three-period cycle, we suggest continuing with some form of aerobic activity and everyday maintenance that includes scaled-down intervals of the stretching and strengthening components of the Triangle of Fitness program.

Warm-Up and Stretching

Whatever your age, the place to start is on the left side of the triangle, with warm-ups and stretching. It's always hard to get into a new habit, so try to pick a convenient time of the day when you are likely to be relaxed and not preoccupied with pressing matters. Once a day is adequate. After a five-minute warm-up period of jogging in place, walking about briskly, or simple limbering exercises, do the following ten stretching exercises. If you are out of shape and your muscles are tight, you may not be able to do all ten comfortably at first. If that's the case, don't try all ten. Do only as many as you can without causing strain or discomfort. You can then gradually work your way to doing all of them within the overall six-week stretching exercise period (give or take a few weeks, depending on your age and physical condition).

Breathing properly is crucial. You should always take a deep breath at the start of an exercise to help deliver oxygen and nutrients to the muscles, and then, as you hold the muscles on stretch, you could count out loud to ensure that you exhale regularly and do not allow the pressure inside your chest cavity to build and raise your blood pressure.

Strengthening

After you have been doing the stretching exercises for six weeks (give or take a few weeks), it is time to move on to the strengthening side of the triangle. One of the biggest mistakes people make at health clubs, or even at home, is to start right off with strengthening exercises, especially on those popular new exercise machines. But muscles that are tight and haven't been prestretched can tear or go into spasm all too easily.

Are strengthening exercises really an essential part of regular fitness? Can we be healthy without them? Perhaps. Mountain climbers and runners are fit, and don't have to lift weights to be good at what they do. Aerobic activities themselves involve inadvertent strengthening of many muscle groups. But clearly there are several advantages. Abdominal strengthening protects the back. Quadriceps strengthening adds stability to the knee and therefore is important to runners. And strengthening certain muscle groups can prepare you for specific sports, such as the shoulder muscles for swimming. Weight exercises for your forearms are good to do during the two or three months before you start playing tennis in the spring, and pulley activities for your arms and shoulders are helpful in preparing you for cross-country skiing.

Having completed your daily warm-up and stretching, do the ten strengthening exercises that follow. Again, depending on your condition and how you feel, you may be able to do only two or three at first; you should then gradually build up over the cycle period. Once you are doing all ten, however, follow up with some abbreviated stretching to cut down on muscle soreness. Don't forget to observe proper breathing techniques. Strengthening exercises can be done three times a week. There is no evidence that daily strengthening is necessary, and a break of a day or two gives the muscles a chance to recoup. But stretching should be continued daily.

If you are about to be engaged in a sport, don't wait too long to begin the strengthening. A sore knee may be caused by weak quadriceps muscles; a painful lower back may be the result of weak abdominals; and a tennis elbow may have its origin in weak forearm muscles.

Aerobic Activity

For the base of the triangle, aerobic activity, there are many alternatives. One of my favorites is walking! In fact, I consider walking to be the best way to ease into aerobics, even if you choose to move on to jogging or some other aerobic sport later on. It's good for your leg muscles, it helps pump blood back to your heart, and it doesn't pound your joints. If done briskly enough, it has true aerobic benefits. It's good for heart attack victims, it stimulates bone metabolism, and it can have a calming effect.

Perhaps you could walk a few blocks in your neighborhood after dinner, or get off the bus sooner on your way to work and walk the rest of the way. Shopping centers and malls can be good for walking. Many modern airports are excellent with their long passageways and corridors. These walking periods could then be lengthened to about twenty or thirty minutes a day. When you are able to cover two miles without too much difficulty, you could then choose three days of the week to pick up your speed substantially.

Walking doesn't cost a thing—except for a good pair of running shoes (make sure they have cushioned heels, a wide toe box, a flexible sole, and a firm "counter" around the heel)—and the proper technique is simplicity itself. You should walk smoothly and easily, letting your arms swing as you move, without exaggeration.

When does walking, or for that matter any vigorous activity, become aerobic? You'll have to monitor your pulse to tell. At the height of or following a good workout, take your pulse—either from your wrist or the carotid artery in your neck, whichever gives the more perceptible beat—over a fifteen-second span, then multiply the result by four to get your pulse rate per minute. What you are aiming for is your own particular "target rate" for maximum body efficiency—that is, the rate beyond which there would be no additional aerobic benefit. This target rate is age-related. You can compute your own by subtracting your age from 220 and taking 75 percent of the difference. For example, if you are sixty years of age, your target rate would be 120 ($220 - 60 = 160 \times .75 = 120$).

When you can sustain your target rate for twenty minutes of activity, you will have become a true "aerobist." However long it takes you to work up to this level, the aerobic "leg" of your fitness-triangle program is not complete until and unless you achieve it. In other words, you will have spent six weeks (give or take) stretching, then six weeks (give or take) strengthening (or you will have started your aerobics with the stretching cycle). If you can then maintain your target rate (over a twenty-minute period) after, say, two to three weeks of aerobic activity, fine, though in this case I would like to see you continue and complete the full six-week period of the program. If, on the other hand, you have not achieved your target rate by gradually intensifying your activity over the full six weeks, you should continue until you do.

Of course, brisk walking is only one type of aerobic activity. Hiking is another of my favorites. If you use hiking for an aerobic activity, be sure you choose an area with good hiking trails. On rocky terrain you have to watch every step, and it will not be easy to maintain your target rate for twenty minutes at a time. If you walk briskly up-hill, the target rate is usually easily reached, so you should enjoy the scenery and not become a nervous wreck trying to take your pulse rate! If you are hiking on hilly terrain, use only the ascent for your aerobic workout. I know of many knee and ankle injuries from walking downhill or, worse still, running downhill—this is very stressful for the knees and ankles. So do not attempt to achieve target rates on the downhill slopes. It is too dangerous. Instead, use the downhill trip as a cooling-off period.

Cross-country skiing is one of the best of all aerobic exercises, especially for people over fifty. If you can walk briskly enough for aerobic benefit, and have no problems with your arms or shoulders, this sport may be an exciting and rewarding challenge for you. Less dangerous than downhill skiing, long-distance skiing, or Nordic as it is sometimes called, provides substantial upper and lower body stretching and strengthening as well as aerobic benefits. If you can walk two or three miles an hour, you can go about twice as fast on the long, narrow skis used in this sport—and burn up to 1,000 calories an hour. What are the advantages of cross-country skiing? There are two, really: first, the torso and upper body extremities are always in action. By using long poles to enhance forward movement, the cross-country skier is actually "walking" on all fours, his arms and shoulders moving as vigorously as his legs. The second advantage involves what is known as the micropause, a moment of relaxation in midstride that allows the muscles to relax and expel waste products without slowing forward motion. This is one of the reasons why muscle and skeletal pain is normally less with cross-country skiing than with jogging or running. There is no jarring of the joints and after a day of skiing across open, gently rising and sloping ground, you are much more likely to experience a pleasing sense of general fatigue. In addition, cross-country skiing is not cumulative in the demands it places on the cardiovascular system. Once you get underway, though your muscles will continue to contract and relax, your cardiac load will probably not increase, and it may even decrease once you have settled into your skiing rhythm.

There are some equipment precautions that you should take when you attempt this sport. The safest types of boots to use in cross-country skiing are those that attach to the skis only at the toes. Because of the substantial upper and lower body movement produced in cross-country skiing, you have to dress carefully and sensibly. Long underwear may be appropriate, depending on the temperature, along with knee socks and knickers below, and shirts and sweaters above. Knickers are particularly important; unlike ski pants and jeans, they do not restrict the rotation of your hips as you move. For women, a firm bra is important because the constant motion of the upper body may have a friction effect on the breasts. There is no way to strengthen breast tissue, so it's a good idea to provide maximum support. For shirts or blouses, cotton is the very best fabric to wear next to your skin; it absorbs moisture easily and dries quickly. A knapsack or waist pack can also be helpful, because it will give you a place to put the layers of clothing you want to remove as you warm up. The knapsack will also allow you to take food—dried fruits or nuts— along if you plan on skiing for any length of time—a very important advantage. When you take a break, make sure you don't cool off too much; this can lead to muscle cramps. Finally, because 80 percent of the body's heat is lost through the head, wearing a woolen hat is advisable.

Many of you, as previously noted, may already be into some recreational sport that is potentially aerobic (including brisk walking or hiking). Perhaps you have kept it up through the stretching and strengthening phases of the program. If so, you may be very close to your target rate by the time you enter the aerobic phase— you may have even achieved it! If close to it, you should intensify your plan and practice until you reach it, then continue through the remainder of the six weeks; if

you have already achieved it, keep it up for the full six weeks. Or, for that matter, however long you wish!

Some sports are more aerobic than others, as shown on the chart on page 38, where we also indicate each sport's musculoskeletal benefits and risks. The choice is yours, and, indeed, you may want to take part in more than one through the aerobic phase. The one important consideration is that, singly or in combination, you practice the activity diligently enough (we recommended, remember, three times a week) and with sufficient intensity to reach your aerobic target rate. Remember, too, to continue your stretching (with warm-up) daily, your strengthening at least three times weekly, and to start every session of aerobic (or potentially aerobic) activity with a five-minute warm-up.

And last, it is important that you finish any and every aerobic session with a cool-down. Most any light activity—walking around briskly, for example—will do if kept up for about five minutes. You can add a little stretching if you'd like to help cut down on the chance of sore muscles after your workout.

An Everyday Maintenance Program

Ideally, from my standpoint, you will want (and be able) to keep up some form of aerobic activity on a regular basis after completing the Triangle of Fitness program. But an aerobic program—without stretching and strengthening—will likely not be enough to maintain your body at an adequate level of fitness. People have often

SPORT	AEROBIC (CARDIOVASCULAR) BENEFITS	MUSCULOSKELETAL BENEFITS	RISKS
Baseball	Low	Shoulder muscle strengthening Forearm muscle strengthening Eye-hand coordination	Rotator cuff tears Hamstring pulls Groin pulls Elbow chips
Cross-country skiing	High	Upper-arm strengthening Chest muscle stretching Hip muscle stretching Calf muscle strengthening	"Tennis" elbow Groin pull
Downhill skiing	High	Coordination and timing Quadriceps strengthening	Fractures Knee ligament injuries Rotator cuff tears
Golf	Without Cart: low With Cart: none	Leg muscle strengthening Hip muscle stretching Shoulder muscle stretching	Golfer's elbow Back muscle spasm Groin pull
Running	High	Leg muscle strengthening Hip muscle stretching	Runner's knee Plantar fasciitis Heel spurs Hip pain
Soccer	High	Quadriceps strengthening Thigh muscle strengthening Stomach muscle strengthening	Quadriceps rupture Knee ligament injuries Groin pull
Squash	High	As with tennis	Eye injuries Wrist sprains As with tennis
Swimming	High	Shoulder muscle strengthening Chest muscle strengthening Thigh muscle strengthening	Neck pain
Tennis	Singles: moderate to high Doubles: low	Eye-hand coordination Forearm muscle strengthening Shoulder stretching, strengthening Leg muscle strengthening	Tennis elbow Achilles tendon rupture Plantaris tendon rupture Hamstring pull Groin pull

asked me what the absolute minimum should be for a daily routine of body maintenance, and what could be safely recommended for most people at any age. I suggest a program that takes between twenty and twenty-five minutes, really quite a reasonable block of time for most of us, and it should include the following:

Warm-ups:	Jogging in place or walking	5 minutes
Stretching:	Hamstrings	5 minutes
	Hip flexors	
	Back extensors	
Strengthening:	Abdominal muscles	5 minutes
	Quadriceps muscles	
Cool-downs:	Jogging in place or walking	5 minutes

Stretching the hamstrings and hip flexors keeps the pelvis from tilting forward and placing extra stress on the lower back area. Stretching the back extensors also helps protect you from back discomfort.

Strengthening of the abdominal muscles is a must. Unlike most other muscle groups, these tend to become loose and slack as the years go by, again straining the lower back area. The quadriceps muscles help stabilize the knee and cut down on the chance of injury.

This daily program will help to keep you fit, and will provide a foundation for those aerobic sports you do choose to continue.

There is a final element in following an exercise program that one might think need not be said, yet it is crucially important. It is best illustrated in my mind by a gentleman who skies with remarkable grace and elegance down the finest slopes in Europe, despite serious wartime injuries to his legs. Many doctors, after seeing his X-rays and examining him, had told him he would never ski again. But he was very determined and committed. Tirelessly, he worked at making every healthy part of his body compensate for the damage, and eventually he succeeded. The lesson? In spite of all the scientific knowledge and clinical experience that physicians use to predict future levels of performance, we see over and over how the human body can respond to exercise and training in the most remarkable ways—especially if the extra ingredients of *determination* and *commitment* are present.

Now that you have a general foundation of fitness and body maintenance, we turn to the large and important subject of the repair and maintenance of specific parts of the body, and the injuries and ailments they can incur, as treated with the techniques of physical medicine. You will discover that many of the same exercises used for maintenance are also used for repair, though in different and special ways. That is the heart of physiatrics. By understanding the workings of your body, you can help maintain it in as fine-tuned a condition as possible throughout your life.

During the first week, begin with five repetitions daily for each stretching exercise. You may add one repetition per week after that, until you can do twelve repetitions comfortably. Remember to inhale at the start of the exercise, then exhale as you hold the muscles on stretch.

STRETCHING

EXERCISE 1

This exercise is designed to stretch the muscles at the back of the neck, muscles that often tighten up during the day because of stress and tension. To begin the exercise, sit on a straight-backed chair with your feet flat on the floor and your arms hanging loosely at your sides. Keep your head level, your neck relaxed. Slowly bring your chin down toward your chest, stopping when you feel tension. Hold that position, breathing regularly, until the tension begins to ease. When it does, bend a bit further; stop when you feel tightness again. Breathe slowly as you wait for the tension to subside, then go further. Hold and breathe at each level and stop when you have gone as far as you can. Hold at this final position for 5 seconds (count to 6) then slowly return to the starting position.

EXERCISE 1

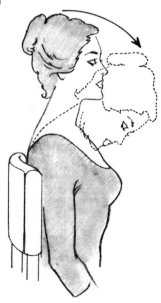

EXERCISE 2

This exercise involves gentle shoulder shrugging and helps stretch the trapezius and rhomboid muscles, which are located in the back of the neck and upper part of the back. Sit in a straight-backed chair with your feet flat on the floor and your hands resting in your lap. Slowly raise your shoulders toward your ears as far as you can without straining. The upward movement may hurt a bit. This sequence should take about 5 seconds (count to 6). Then let your shoulders slowly return to their normal position. Be sure to relax completely (count to 5) between each repetition and to breathe regularly as you do the exercise.

EXERCISE 2

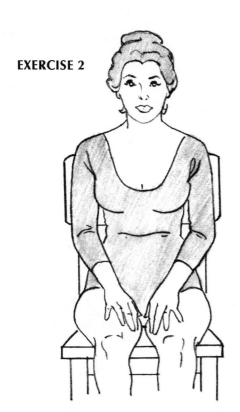 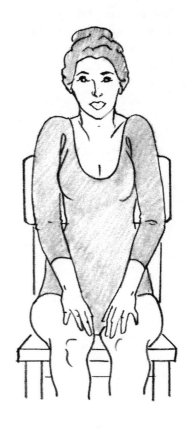

EXERCISE 3

This exercise will stretch muscles in the front and rear of your shoulders and upper back. Sit in a straight-backed chair with your feet flat on the floor. Place the tips of your fingers on your shoulders—right hand on right shoulder, left hand on left shoulder. Now, keeping your hands in place, slowly bring your elbows together, at shoulder level, and try to touch them in front of your chin. Stop when you feel tension, hold the position and breathe regularly until tension subsides, then continue moving elbows together until you again feel tension; hold, breathe regularly, and wait for the tension to subside. Don't force it. If you can, touch your elbows, hold for 5 seconds, then return to starting position and relax. Next, bring your elbows back, opening your rib cage, until you feel tension in your shoulder muscles. Again, hold and breathe until tension diminishes, then return to starting position and relax.

EXERCISE 3

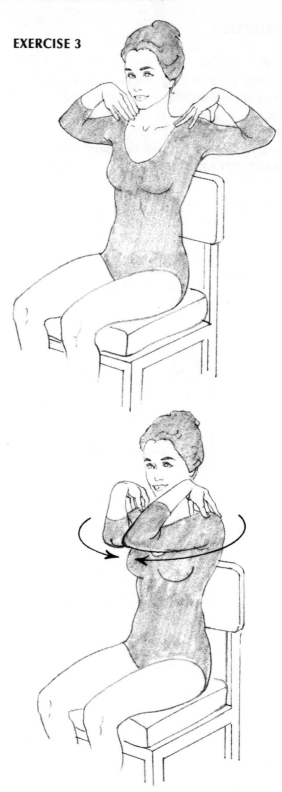

EXERCISE 4

This exercise will stretch your upper and lower back extensor muscles. Sit in a straight-backed chair with your feet flat on the floor, your knees shoulder-width apart, and your hands hanging loosely at your sides or between your knees. First tuck your chin toward your chest, then slowly roll down, bringing your shoulders toward your knees. Do not strain or bounce. Hold this position for 5 seconds (count to 6). Tighten your abdominal muscles, squeeze your buttocks together, and return to the starting position by slowly unrolling, first your lower back, then your shoulders, and lastly your head. Relax. Remember to exhale when rolling down, and to inhale on the way up.

EXERCISE 4

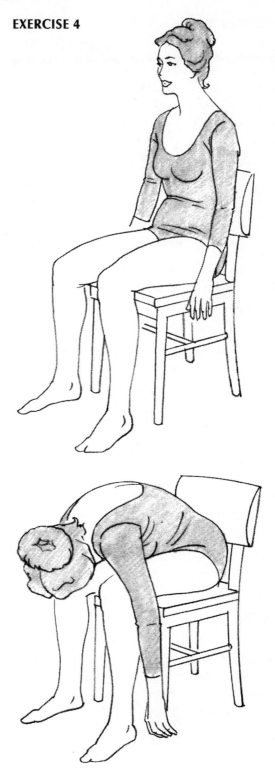

EXERCISE 5

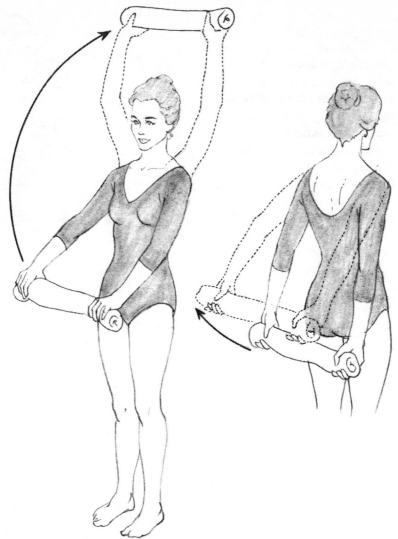

EXERCISE 5

This exercise is twofold and will help loosen muscles in both your back and chest. Do not force it; stop, breathe, and wait for tension to subside. To start, stand upright with your feet about 6 inches apart, arms straight in front of your body. Holding a rolled towel in your hands, slowly bring it up and over your head, then back toward your neck and upper back. Keep your arms straight. Do not arch your back and do not strain. Hold this position, breathing regularly, and wait for tension to subside. Slowly return to starting position and relax. The second starting position is the same as the first except you're holding the towel behind you. Gently raise your arms up and away from your body as far as you can without straining. Keep your arms straight. Hold this position, breathing regularly, and wait for the tension to subside. Slowly return to the starting position and relax.

EXERCISE 6

For this hip flexor stretch, lie on your back near the end of a bed. Bend your knees and place your feet flat at the edge of the mattress. Bring one knee up toward your chest and hold it firmly in place by clasping your hands around the lower part of the leg. Lower the other leg so that your knee bends over the edge of the mattress and hangs free. Hold this stretch position for 15 to 30 seconds. Be sure to breathe regularly throughout the exercise. Return to the starting position and relax, then repeat with the other leg.

EXERCISE 6

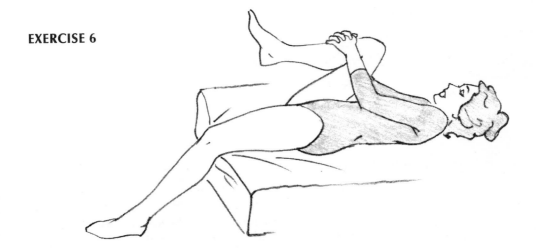

EXERCISE 7

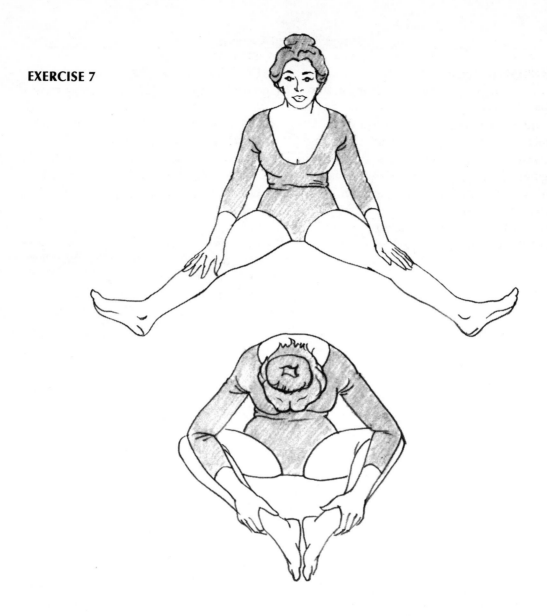

EXERCISE 7

This exercise will stretch your hip adductor muscles—the muscles that bring your legs together. Sit on the floor with your legs outstretched in a V position. Bend your knees and move your feet in toward your body until the soles of your feet come together. Place your hands on your ankles and bend over slightly so that your elbows rest on the inside of your knees. Slowly press down with your elbows, gradually pushing your knees toward the floor. Breathe regularly, hold 15 to 30 seconds, and wait until tension subsides. Continue the downward pressure until the next point of tension and hold for 15 to 30 seconds, breathing regularly. Do not force the movement or bounce. When you have gone as far as you can, slowly return to the starting position and relax.

46

EXERCISE 8

This exercise will stretch your hamstrings—the muscles in the back of your upper leg. Lie on your back with your arms relaxed at your side, knees bent, feet slightly apart and flat on the floor. Slowly push the small of your back into the floor while bringing your right knee toward your chest, with foot flexed. Slowly straighten the right leg (you may have to lower your leg to achieve this) until you feel tension in the back of the leg, then stop, breathe regularly, and wait for tension to subside. Continue to the next friction point until you reach the position in which the leg is most comfortable and fully extended. Hold for 15 to 30 seconds, then relax for 10 seconds (count to 12). Make sure that all tension leaves your muscles. Repeat the exercise with your other leg.

EXERCISE 8

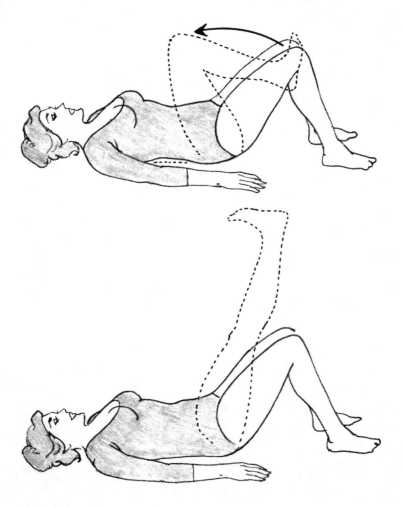

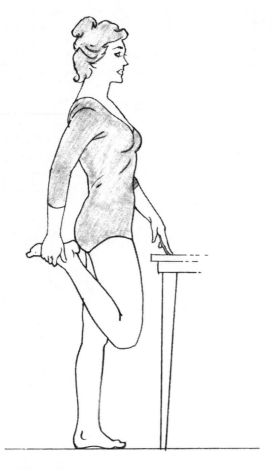

EXERCISE 9

This is a runner's exercise, one that is designed to stretch your quadriceps—the muscle in the front of your upper leg. Stand with one hand lightly touching a wall or the edge of a table for balance; with your other hand, grab your foot (right hand, right leg; left hand, left leg) and gently ease your heel up toward your buttock without straining. Stop when you feel tension, breathe regularly until the pull subsides, then continue until your heel is as close to your buttock as possible without pain or excessive tension. Do not arch your back. Hold for 15 to 30 seconds, then relax completely, letting all tension leave the muscle.

EXERCISE 10

This is another runner's exercise that will stretch your calf muscles. Stand about 18 to 24 inches from a wall, feet together and flat on the floor; press your palms against the wall at shoulder height. Bend your elbows and lean your upper body into the wall. Be sure to keep your heels flat on the floor and your knees straight. You will feel tension in your calf muscles at the back of your legs. Do not arch your back. Hold your position at the point of tension, breathing regularly, and wait for tension to subside (15 to 20 seconds). Relax completely for 10 seconds (count to 12).

One of the valuable aspects of this ten-exercise program is that you can take it apart and use certain exercises at certain times. For instance, if you are outside and feel like going for a walk or run, you can do the last three to loosen your major lower-leg muscles groups—hamstrings, quadriceps, and calf muscles. The full program can also function as a complete stretching workout as well as a preparation for the strengthening exercises.

STRENGTHENING

EXERCISE 1

There are only two facial muscles that lend themselves to strengthening by exercise; both are in the lower portion of your face. By working to strengthen them, you'll reduce sagging in the area. The first part of the exercise is simple and common: a smile, but a deep one that forces your cheeks back—hold for 5 seconds (count to 6). Relax for 4 seconds (count to 5). The second part of the exercise is designed to strengthen your chin muscle. Instead of a smile, produce a grimace; use a mirror to ensure that the line of your expression is downward, as shown in the illustration. Hold for 5 seconds (count to 6) and then relax for 4 seconds (count to 5). Do 8 to 10 repetitions of each part twice a day, morning and night.

EXERCISE 1

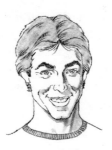

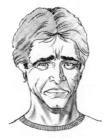

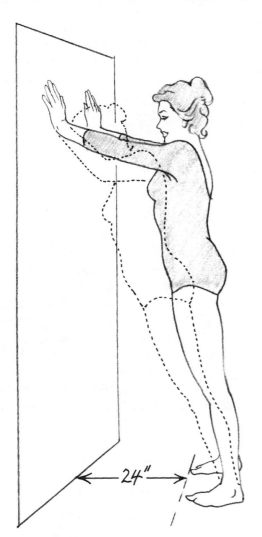

EXERCISE 10

EXERCISE 2

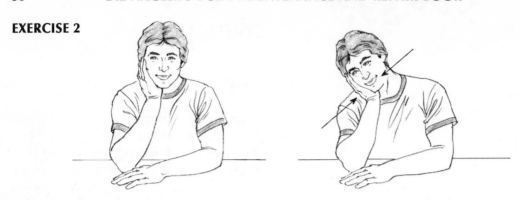

EXERCISE 2

This neck muscle–strengthening exercise is designed to build up the sterno-cleido-mastoid muscle, which turns the neck. Sit in a straight-backed chair with your feet flat on the floor and your elbows resting on a table. Place your right hand on the right side of your face. Push your head against the resistance of your hand and hold for 5 seconds (count to 6). Relax until all tension leaves your muscles, then work the other side of your neck in the same way. Neck muscles tighten up easily, so exercise gently and build strength gradually. Start off doing 3 or 4 repetitions on each side, then begin adding one repetition every other day until you reach 12 a day. Remember: It's important not to hold your breath while exercising.

EXERCISE 3

This exercise is designed to build up the strength of your upper back. Lie on your stomach with a firm pillow under your lower abdomen. Hook your feet or ankles under the edge of a couch or heavy chair. Clasp your hands behind your neck and raise your upper body from the floor. Hold this position for 5 seconds (count to 6), then slowly return to the original prone position. Start with 3 repetitions and add one every other day until you can do 12. If you have any back or shoulder problems, you should consult your doctor before attempting this exercise.

EXERCISE 3

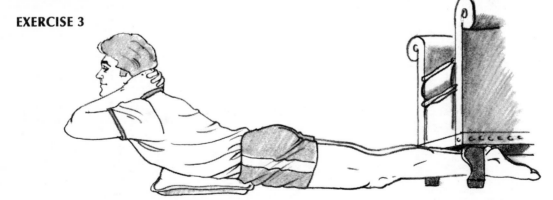

EXERCISE 4

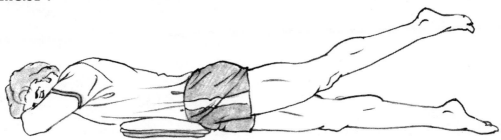

EXERCISE 4

This exercise is similar to the preceding one, except that it is structured to increase lower back and buttock strength. Lie on your stomach with a pillow under your lower abdomen and rest your head on your arms or clasp the legs of a heavy chair or couch. Raise one leg at a time with toes pointed and without bending knee and hold for 5 seconds (count to 6). Relax. Start with 3 repetitions and work up to 12. Remember to breathe normally while exercising. If you have any back problems, you should consult your doctor before attempting this exercise.

EXERCISE 5

This is a relatively simple exercise but a very important one. It will build up your buttock and hip extensor muscles, which help to hold your back and hips in line. To begin, lie on your stomach with a pillow under your abdomen. Squeeze your buttocks together tightly and hold for 5 seconds (count to 6). Relax for 4 seconds (count to 5) and repeat 3 times to start working up to 12 repetitions. If you have difficulty contracting your buttocks, use your hands to gently squeeze them together. You should be able to feel the buttock muscles contract.

EXERCISE 5

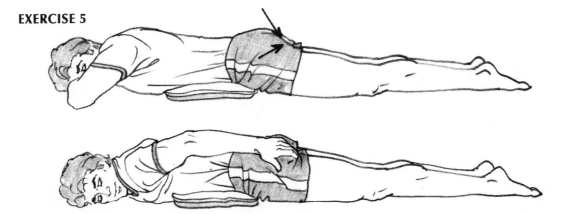

EXERCISE 6, 7, 8

Push-ups are a common enough exercise, but they can be demanding if you haven't done them for years. For this reason, I'm including three kinds of push-ups, arranged in increasing order of difficulty. The first is a wall push-up. Stand about 18 inches from a wall with your arms ex- tended straight in front of your body; do a push-up against the wall by bending your arms at the elbows, moving your body in and out. Keep your back straight and do each repetition slowly, consuming at least 5 seconds (count to 6). Start with 3 or 4 repe- titions and try to work up to 15. Relax be- tween repetitions. After you can do 15 wall push-ups easily, you are ready to switch to

EXERCISE 6

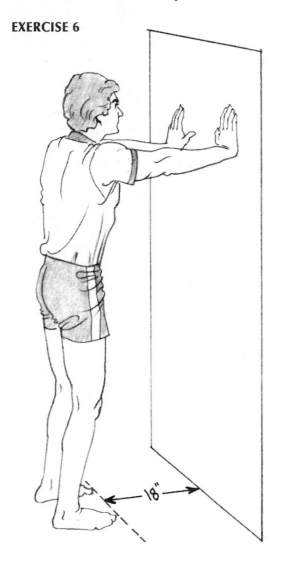
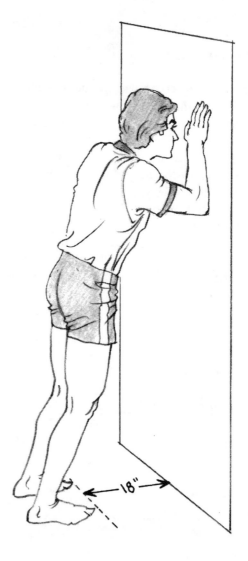

EXERCISE 7

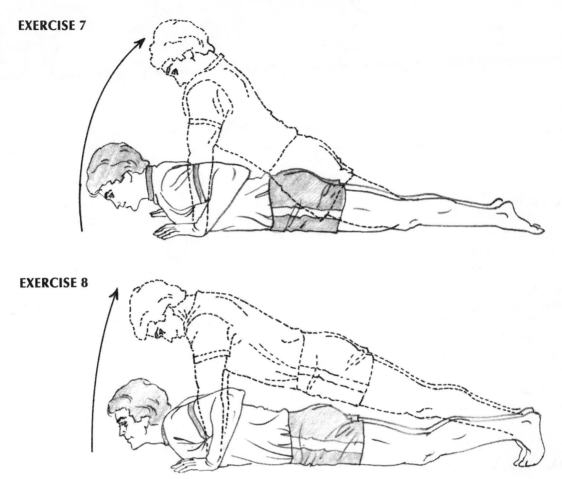

EXERCISE 8

the bent-knee version of the exercise. Lie prone on the floor; place your hands, palms down, beneath your shoulders; and push against the floor with enough force to lift your upper body from shoulders to knees. Hold for 5 seconds (count to 6), then slowly lower your body to the floor and relax. Try for 1 or 2 repetitions at first, slowly increasing to 15. When you can do 15 bent-knee push-ups easily, you're ready to switch to the full push-up. This third type begins in the same fashion as the bent-knee, but now you lift your whole body so that only your hands and toes are supporting your weight. Your toes should be pointed down into the floor, and you should push up slowly in one continuing movement. Keep your shoulders and spine in a straight line. Hold for five seconds (count to 6), then return to the floor and relax. Raise your body again. Start with 3 push-ups and build to 15.

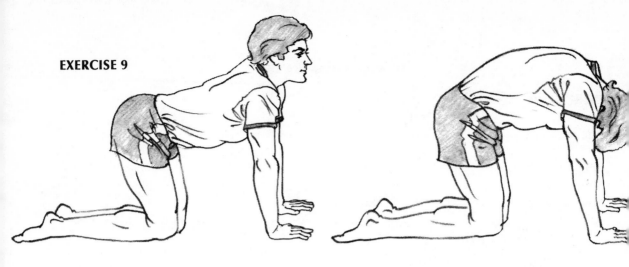

EXERCISE 9

EXERCISE 9

Your abdominal muscles are one of the most important muscle groups in your body, but they can be difficult to strengthen, especially if you haven't exercised in a long time. Therefore, I am including a number of variations (this and the next three exercises), beginning with the easiest and working up in difficulty. When you can do 15 of any of these exercises easily, you're ready to go on to the next level of difficulty.

The easiest way to strengthen your abdominals is to perform an exercise known as a cat back. Get down on your hands and knees (hands under shoulders, knees under hips). Inhale, and then, as you exhale, drop your head and draw your abdominal muscles up into your body. Hold for 5 seconds (count to 6), then relax for 4 seconds (count to 5). Begin this exercise with a small number of repetitions, 3 to 5, and gradually work up to 15.

EXERCISE 10

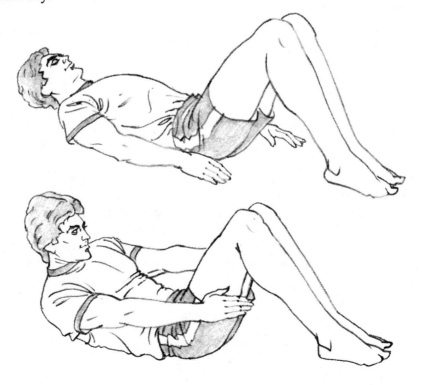

EXERCISE 10

The second type is a sit-up known as the half sit-up. Lie on your back with your arms at your sides and your knees bent. Slowly curl your head, upper back, and arms as far off the floor as you can without straining—at first, you should simply come up gradually into a half sit-up position—then uncurl your body back to the floor. After a few days, you may find yourself able to hold the up position for 5 seconds (count to 6), then drop back and rest for 4 seconds (count to 5). Start with a few repetitions, then gradually increase the number to 15 without straining. When you can do 15, you're ready for the full sit-up.

EXERCISE 11

EXERCISE 11

This exercise is done in the same position as the half sit-up, only this time when you sit up you bring your arms up so that they extend beyond your knees and your forehead comes as close as possible to your kneecaps. If you want to increase the effectiveness of this exercise, do the up and down sequences as slowly as possible; try to consume 5 seconds (count to 6) on the way up and the same coming down. To increase the degree of difficulty you can make a number of changes, as described in the next exercise.

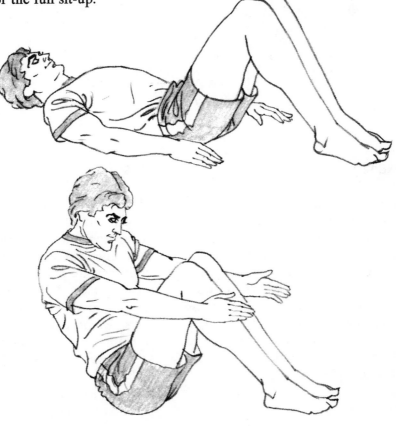

EXERCISE 12

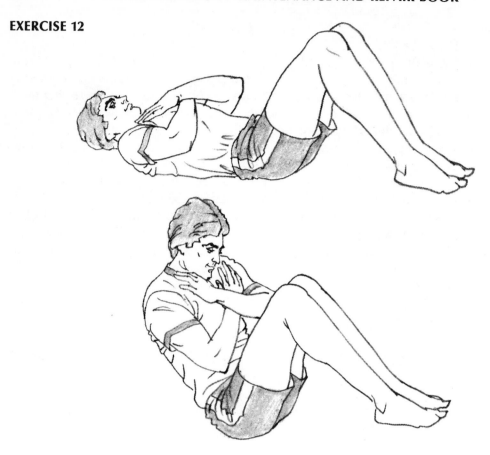

EXERCISE 12

Instead of extending your arms in a forward position, clasp them on your chest as shown in the illustration above. After doing sit-ups in this fashion, you can increase the difficulty again by clasping your hands behind your neck. And if you want to increase the effectiveness of the exercise even more, hold a 2- or 3-pound weight behind your neck, or attach weights to your upper arms. Be careful not to strain the neck and upper back area.

EXERCISE 13

This is a rigorous test of your abdominal muscles. Install a bar across a door frame. Hang from the bar with elbows straight, then raise your legs straight in front of you until they are parallel to the floor. Hold 5 seconds, then slowly lower your legs and relax. You should work up to 15 repetitions. Eventually, you may increase the strength of your abdominal muscles to such a level that you can bring your legs up higher and hold for 5 seconds. As you bring the legs up from the vertical position, be sure to exhale.

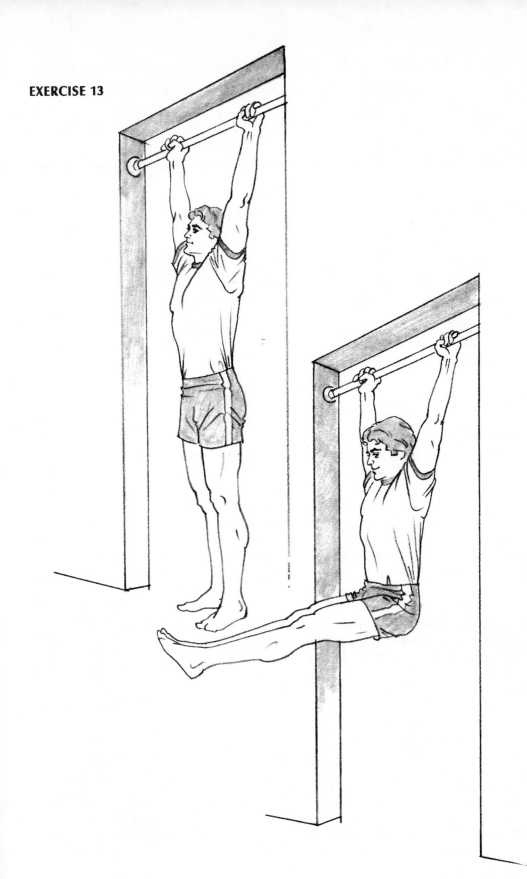

EXERCISE 14

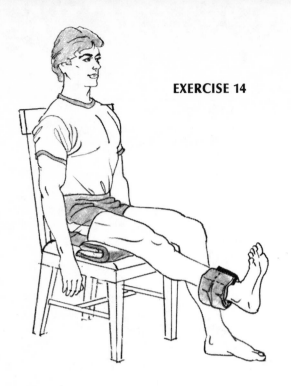

EXERCISE 14

This exercise is designed to strengthen your quadriceps. Start by sitting in a straight-backed chair with a towel under your right thigh and a 3- or 4-pound weight on your ankle. Raise your lower leg until it is in a straight line with the rest of your leg. Hold 5 seconds (count to 6). Slowly return to the starting position and relax. Do 6 or 8 repetitions and slowly build up to 12. You can then increase the weight by a pound or two and, dropping back to 8 repetitions, work up to 12 again. You may keep adding weights until you have reached 10 to 15 pounds. Be sure to exercise both legs equally.

EXERCISE 15

This exercise will strengthen your hip abductor muscles—the muscles that move your leg out to the side. Place a 2- to 3-pound weight around your left ankle. Lie on your right side and, keeping your bottom leg slightly bent and your top leg perfectly straight, slowly lift your left leg straight up, as far as possible. Do not bend at the hip, either to the front or rear. Keep the kneecap of your left leg facing forward and the leg in a straight line from your body. Hold this position while counting out loud to 6 (5 seconds). Slowly lower your leg to the starting position and relax for 4 seconds (count to 5). Start with 8 repetitions and increase to 12. When you can do 12 easily, increase the weight by a pound, drop down to 8 repetitions, and build up to 12 again. You may keep adding weights until you have reached 12 repetitions with 10 to 15 pounds. Follow the same sequence with your right leg, lying on your left side.

EXERCISE 15

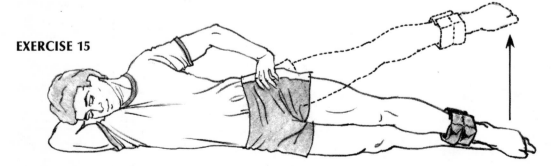

EXERCISE 16

This exercise will strengthen the large and important muscle in your calf, the gastrocnemius muscle. Stand with feet flat on the floor and your hands resting on a sturdy surface to help you maintain your balance. Slowly raise your heels until you are standing on your toes, as in the illustration.

Hold this position for 5 seconds (count to 6), then slowly lower your heels down to the floor. Relax. Start off with 8 repetitions and build to 12. At first, do this exercise with your weight equally distributed over both feet; build up strength in both legs before attempting the exercise with just one foot.

EXERCISE 16

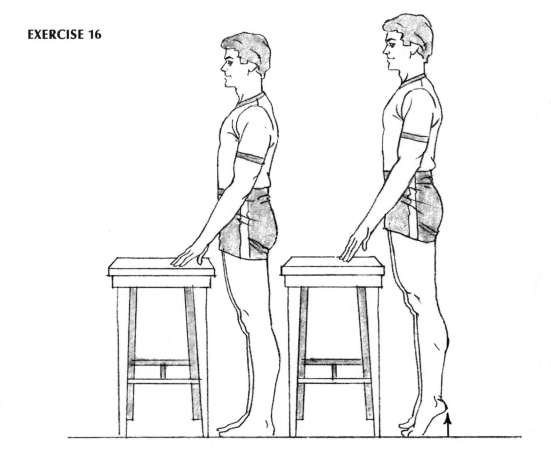

PART TWO

YOUR BODY FROM A TO Z:
An Encyclopedia of Repair and Maintenance

ACHES AND PAINS

Many of us take it for granted that we will never be bothered by aches and pains, until one day we wake up and everything from head to toe seems to ache. We find our energy levels low, and the value of sleep becomes uncertain.

As we get older, especially if we tend to ignore the condition of our muscles, these aches and pains may become so ever-present that they actually affect the quality of life. Seldom can they be explained by laboratory studies or X-rays. If you are around sixty or sixty-five, the probability is very high that you will have some abnormalities of your bony spinal structures, and these will show up on an X-ray. Eighty-seven percent of people over age sixty will have such findings in the neck or cervical spine, but not all will experience pain. By the same token, many others will experience pain but won't show any spinal abnormalities. This is because the discomfort is coming primarily from the muscles.

Why do our muscles start to ache as we get older? Over the years, we tend to become less active. If we don't make a point of exercising regularly, we lose some of our muscle mass. The fine network of blood vessels supplying the muscles becomes "unemployed," and some of the capillaries actually shut down. The ongoing process of fuel delivery and removal of waste prod-

ucts that normally occurs between blood vessel and muscle becomes less efficient. Waste products accumulate and we are left with a feeling of soreness. In addition, the process of aging makes our muscles less elastic, so if we don't exercise and keep them moving they tend to tighten up.

If you don't care for your muscles with daily or at least frequent regular exercise, and you make some sudden increased demands on them, they will hurt. Take swimming. Youngsters can jump into the water and start swimming at high speed immediately because their muscles are young and active and their blood supply is adequate. But if you are older, and even if you are a good swimmer, your muscles have to loosen up before you can get going. Your less efficient blood supply mechanism will not be adequate to meet the sudden demand for oxygen to drive the muscles, which themselves will be weak and stiff from insufficient use.

A younger person can have aches and pains, too. But this usually occurs after some especially strenuous activity, overtaxing even for a basically sound muscle-blood system. Some tiny microtears may then occur throughout the stressed muscle with minute amounts of bleeding. And again, the blood vessel network may not have been able to keep up with the job of removing a larger-than-usual accumulation of waste products. This is what happens with a charley horse (nowadays called DOMT, delayed onset muscle tension). In a younger person, healing will take place very quickly, and after a few days he or she can perform the same kind of activity without incurring any pain. For the older person with sufficient determination and a regular schedule of exercise, improvement can be brought about because muscles are *trainable*. They can be loosened and then strengthened, thus becoming more efficient and less prone to injury. For more information you can consult the "charley horse" section.

It would be best, of course, if daily aches and pains could be prevented in the first place. The way to do this is to keep your muscles strong and limber through daily exercise. The fringe benefits are enormous. Not only will your aches and pains abate, but your overall mobility will improve. This is because of another aspect of the aging process involving joints, in which smooth cartilage becomes roughened and less efficient as a joint-bearing mechanism. Strong and stretched muscles will keep the joints moving smoothly. They will also protect the joints by decreasing the stress exerted on them. You will feel more vigorous and energetic, and your muscles and blood supply will be in a state of readiness for increased demands. It has even been shown in some long-range studies that daily exercise can actually *postpone* the aging effect on the joints by about ten years.

Taken together, all these benefits constitute a powerful argument for exercising your aches and pains away. You should, however, have some medical guidance in assessing your particular situation and in structuring an individualized exercise pro-

gram. Aches and pains can signal an underlying disease process that needs a special approach. I will tell you about two such conditions.

The first is called polymyalgia rheumatica. It is an illness that rarely appears before the age of fifty or so, through after that it gradually becomes more common. Its symptoms include aches and pains in the joints and muscles—especially those of the neck and shoulders—headaches, fatigue, loss of appetite, weight loss, and a feeling of illness. This time there *is* a relatively simple test that can be helpful in pointing toward a specific diagnosis. It is known as ESR, or "sed rate" (for erythrocyte sedimentation rate), and it measures the rate at which red blood cells separate from the blood plasma when traveling down a narrow glass column. Sed rates can be high in a number of conditions, among them polymyalgia rheumatica. A biopsy of one of the arteries in your temple may also be required to determine whether inflammation has occurred due to the disease. Making the correct diagnosis is important because the disease is progressive and, if left untreated, can produce severe headaches, even blindness. So, if aches, pains, fatigue, and weight loss trouble you, you should see your doctor and have a sed rate done. Treatment, usually effective, involves the ingestion of small doses of steroids.

The second problem that can be masked by aches and pains and generalized fatigue is known as fibromyositis. For years, people with this condition were thought to be suffering from depression, with their physical symptoms diagnosed simply as an expression of their emotional state. In the last decade, however, this view has changed, and fibromyositis is now better defined and more fully accepted. A typical complaint from a patient with the problem runs like this: "Doctor, I'm always tired. I wake up in the morning more tired than when I went to bed. My neck and shoulders, hips, and knees hurt me the most." This may sound like plain old aches and pains, but very often when I examine such patients, most of them likely to be in their forties, I find small subcutaneous knots or nodules, usually clustered in groups of ten or twelve, in the very areas of complaint. Recent studies have also shown that fibromyositis patients often have irregular brain wave patterns during periods of dream sleep, which suggests that they do not sleep in the same way the rest of us do, and explains why they are constantly tired. The stories such patients tell are usually quite similar. The patients were active when they were younger. Then the demands of business and home life cut down on their other activities. Whenever they tried to return to regular exercise, everything seemed to hurt. Finally, they lost interest in exercise and stopped altogether. Many of these patients will have seen a number of physicians and taken a variety of medications.

Perhaps the most helpful thing a physician can do for these patients is to tell them they have a specific medical condition and their problems do not exist exclusively in their minds. Treatment is difficult and requires emotional support and clear guidance as much as anything else. The painful nodules can be massaged away, a structured exercise program can help loosen and strengthen unused muscles, and medication may help to improve the restorative function of sleep. Ultimately, such pa-

tients, with help and support, will move into regular physical activity on their own. Even simple walking or jogging several times a week can be enough to reestablish activity and improve muscle tone. Once this happens, victims of this debilitating condition begin to lose their fear of physical activity, and their chances for full recovery become good.

A diagnosis of fibromyositis is not accepted by all physicians, but I do believe that the physical evidence and the clinical response I have observed over the years support this diagnosis at least as well as many other well-recognized disease entities in medicine. Fibromyositis is not an intractable condition and should never be written off as unresponsive to medical treatment. It is not easy to return someone with fibromyositis to full function, but it can be done.

ACHILLES TENDON

Capable of bearing over a half ton of weight, the heavy tendon that connects the calf muscle to the heel bone is vulnerable to two types of damage. The first type of damage is an inflammation, or Achilles tendinitis, which develops gradually from overuse. The second is rupture, which may occur in the competitive athlete as the result of a quick start and the powerful contraction of the calf muscle, or in the weekend sports enthusiast whose calf muscle is less conditioned and inadequately stretched before a workout.

An inflamed Achilles tendon will start to

settle down if you apply ice to it twice a day for 4 or 5 minutes at a time (see Cold and Heat Treatments, page 91) and eliminate athletic activities (except swimming) for 4 to 6 weeks.

If you rupture your Achilles tendon you'll feel a pop in the back of your leg between your lower calf and heel (you may also lose your balance and fall), rather as if someone has whacked you there with the edge of a tennis racquet. Though the pain may not be excessive, you'll find walking difficult, and most likely possible only with a limp. Soon enough you'll realize that you've suffered more than a minor injury and will seek medical treatment.

If you were to arrive at my office, I'd first listen very carefully to your story and then ask you to rise gently on your toes. If you couldn't do this, I'd have you lie on your stomach and bend the knee of your injured leg. If I then pressed on both sides of your calf and your foot didn't move upward slightly, I'd know that your Achilles tendon had been ruptured. What I would have performed on you is called the Thompson test.

There are two courses of treatment available at this point. One is for an orthopedist to put your ankle and leg in a cast and give the fibers of the torn tendon time to reattach; the other is for him to stitch the injured fibers back together. On the whole, I favor the second approach, for it ensures a firm tendon connection.

The decision as to whether you should be treated with a leg cast only, or with surgical intervention first and a leg cast afterward, depends very much on the degree of rupture and on your age. If you have an incomplete rupture, the muscles that enable you to move your foot during the Thompson test may be less effective, but there will still be some motion. In such a situation the leg cast may suffice. If the rupture is complete, it means the upper part of the tendon is completely separated from the muscle, and in these cases especially I feel surgical repair is preferable. If you plan to engage in athletic activity and have a vigorous life-style, you should also definitely have the surgery. If, however, you have reached an age where you do not plan to engage in any strenuous athletic activities, you would probably do just as well with only a leg cast.

In either case, you'll have to wear a cast for six to eight weeks and, when the cast is removed, be prepared to stretch and strengthen your calf muscles (tendons don't stretch, only muscles do).

The following are specific therapeutic exercises to be performed following the removal of the cast. They are designed to stretch and strengthen the calf muscles after your ruptured Achilles tendon has healed, and should be done twice a day. Stretching is important because the fibers in your calf muscles will have shortened as they healed. Be careful not to overstretch; this can rerupture fibers, especially in the early stages of the healing process. Be sure to breathe regularly while doing the exercises, and to relax completely between repetitions. Do not do the fourth or fifth exercise before you can do 15 repetitions of the third with 3 pounds.

EXERCISE 1

Sit on the floor, back against the wall, and extend your legs in front of you, ankles together. Reach forward and hook a rolled towel around the balls of your feet. Keeping your knees straight, pull back firmly on the towel until you feel tension in the back of your lower legs. Hold for 15 seconds (count to 18), then release. Relax for 10 seconds (count to 12) or until you feel that all of the tension has left the muscle. Do 5 or 6 repetitions.

EXERCISE 1

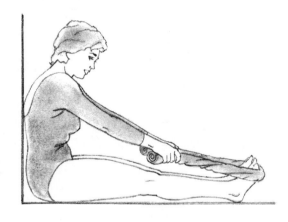

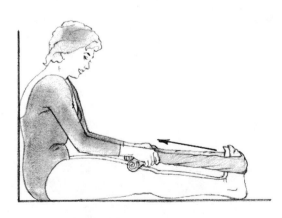

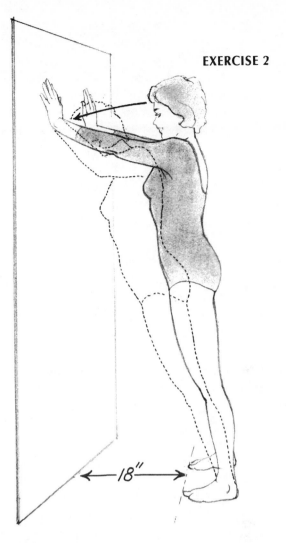

EXERCISE 2

This is a traditional runner's exercise, and you have probably seen people doing it. Stand about 18 to 24 inches from a wall, feet together and heels flat on the floor; press your palms against the wall. Bend your elbows and lean your upper body into the wall. Be sure to keep your heels on the floor and your knees straight. Do not arch your back. You will feel the pull at the back of your legs. Hold for 15 seconds (count to 18), then release. Relax for 10 seconds (count to 12) or until you feel that all of the tension has left the muscle. Do 5 or 6 repetitions.

EXERCISE 3

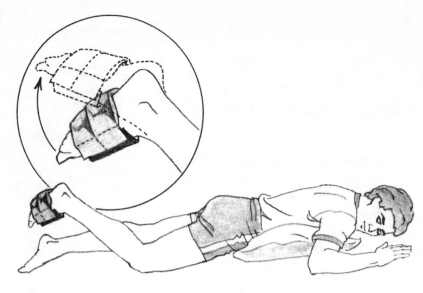

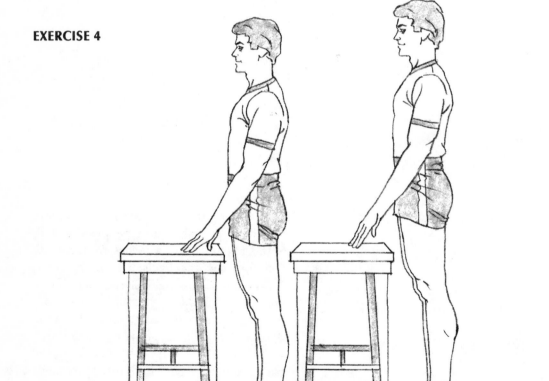

EXERCISE 4

EXERCISE 3

This exercise is designed to strengthen the calf, or gastrocnemius, muscle. Lie on your stomach with a pillow under your abdomen and weights strapped to the toes of your injured foot. Bend the knee and lift the leg to a 45-degree angle. From this starting position, point your toes toward the ceiling and hold for 5 seconds (count to 6). Drop your toes, but not your leg, and relax for 3 seconds (count to 4). Start off using a weight that you can comfortably lift 8 times (for most adults, 1 or 2 pounds). When you can do 12 repetitions easily, add a pound and drop down to 8 repetitions. Your eventual goal is to do 12 repetitions with 3 or 4 pounds.

EXERCISE 4

Here is another exercise designed to strengthen the gastrocnemius muscle. Stand with feet flat on the floor and your hands resting on a sturdy table to help you maintain your balance. Slowly raise your heels until you are standing on your toes. Hold for 5 seconds (count to 6), then lower your heels and relax until all of the tension has left the muscle. Start off doing 15 repetitions with your body weight distributed equally over both feet. Build up strength in both legs before attempting this with just the injured leg. Continue using a table to balance yourself. When you can exercise your injured leg alone, start with 5 repetitions, adding one repetition a day until you reach a maximum of 15.

EXERCISE 5

Superstretch. Stand 18 to 24 inches from a wall with your feet together; place your palms against the wall. Bend your elbows and lean your upper body into the wall. Keep your heels on the floor and your knees straight. Do not arch your back. You will feel the pull at the back of your legs. Put the heel of the uninjured leg above the kneecap of the injured one and press against it. You will feel an additional stretch in the calf muscle. You may gradually increase the duration of the stretch from 5 to 15 seconds.

EXERCISE 5

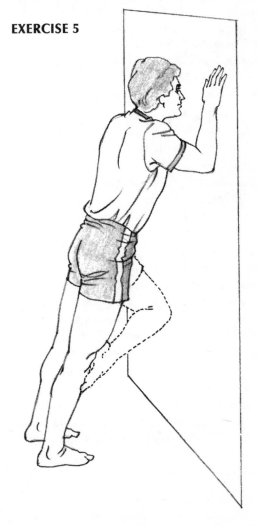

ACUPUNCTURE FOR PAIN RELIEF

Acupuncture has been with man for a long time. It has been used in China for thousands of years, along with herbal medicine, for the control of pain and the treatment of many illnesses. Yet it was not until the age of television and President Nixon's trip to China that acupuncture began to receive widespread attention in the United States.

The practice of acupuncture is based on the theory of energy-flow pathways in the body. Along such postulated pathways or "meridians" lie many acupuncture "points" on the skin, each about three millimeters in diameter. By inserting a fine needle into the skin at one of these points, and twirling it in a certain way, an acupuncturist is theoretically trying to alter the energy flow of a disturbed pattern. (It is my understanding that acupuncture points were discovered empirically by Eastern health practitioners who found that they were able to provide pain relief and other beneficial results by *pressing* on certain areas of the body; only later was the insertion of needles found to be more effective.)

The acupuncture effect cannot be explained by current concepts of neurophysiology and the physiology of pain. Meridians do not correspond to nerve-fiber pathways, and the increased levels of endorphins—the body's own natural painkillers—that are found after acupuncture treatments are also found after other invasive procedures, and do not explain the sometimes long-lasting relief some people experience. Interestingly enough, 70 percent of acupuncture points are in the same location as commonly detected muscular trigger points (see Trigger Points). The connection between the two, however, is not understood.

In addition to regular needle acupuncture, it is also possible to have *electro-acupuncture*, which is based on the same principles but achieved by administering a very mild electrical current, in the 25 to 200 microampere range, through the needle. And then there is *acupressure,* which, as mentioned, uses no needles at all and simply involves pressing down on acupuncture points without penetrating the skin. This is something you can do yourself, unlike acupuncture, which requires the expertise of a skilled practitioner.

I do believe that acupuncture has a definite place in medicine and deserves to be the focus of continuing intensive research efforts. Any technique that can offer pain relief without side effects is highly worthwhile! Unfortunately, we don't yet understand how it works, and why it works on some people and not on others. If you have continuing musculoskeletal pain from a well-established medical illness, and have not obtained significant pain relief from other forms of indicated medical treatment, there is no reason not to give acupuncture a try. You should have it done by physicians who have been specially trained in it.

ANATOMICAL TERMS

Physiatrists and other physicians use specific terms to describe the position and motions of different parts of the body. Unless you know at least the principal terms, you will not be able to correctly perform the exercises you are likely to come across at health clubs or in fitness magazines and in the literature your doctor may give you.

The basic body position from which these anatomical terms are derived consists of an upright body facing forward with the arms at the sides and the palms turned forward. Deviations from this basic position are given special names. For instance, *abduction* is the movement of a limb away from the center of the body. Your shoulder is "abducting" when you move your arm straight out to the side and up, as though you were raising your hand in class. We also talk frequently about abducting the hip, which is what you do when you are lying on your side and raise the upper leg as far as you can toward the ceiling.

The opposite of abduction is *adduction*—that is, the movement of a limb toward or across the center of the body. If you are standing and talking to someone, and you cross one leg in front of the other to be more comfortable, you are adducting your hip. Or, if you are sitting at a desk and you reach across your body with your right arm to answer a phone placed on the left side of the desk, you are adducting your shoulder.

"Flexion" and "extension" are two terms you hear frequently. Conceptually, *flexion* refers to narrowing the angle of a joint. For instance, if you "flex your muscles" in order to show off the bulge of the biceps muscle in your upper arm, you are really bending or flexing your elbow joint, bringing it from a position of approximately 180 degrees to a position of approximately 90 degrees. When you lean forward, you are bending or flexing your trunk or upper body. If you bring your chin to your chest, you are flexing your neck. While sitting in a chair with your feet on the floor, both your hips and knees are flexed, as they are when you lie on your back and bring your knees to your chest.

Extension is the opposite of flexion. It refers to increasing the angle of a joint. If you straighten your arm or knee, you are extending your elbow and knee joints. If you take a step backward, you have just extended your hip. If you look up at the ceiling, or arch your back, you are extending your neck and back with the help of your neck and back extensor muscles. If you arch your back *too* much, you are *hyperextending* it.

It may be hard to remember the difference between wrist flexion and extension, because either way you are bending your wrist and changing the angle in relation to the arm. If you have ever had tennis elbow, or are concerned about developing it, you will appreciate the fact that your wrist extensor muscles, which attach at the outer side of your elbow, are responsible for the problem. If you rest the flat side of your forearm on a table and bring your wrist back, it is in extension. If you curl the wrist down in the other direction, it is in flexion.

It gets even more complicated with the ankle. You might expect that the up and down motions of the ankle would simply be called extension and flexion, as they are in the wrist. However, ankle terms are related to the surfaces of the foot: the top or instep of the foot is the "dorsum," and moving the ankle so that the toes point up is *dorsiflexion*. It is analagous to extending the wrist, but you won't hear anyone talking about "ankle extension." (Sometimes you will hear people use the term dorsiflexion when talking about wrist extension. It is not a bad term as such—it does describe the motion of bending your wrist back—but I prefer "wrist extension" to avoid confusion.) The bottom or sole of the foot is its "plantar" surface. When you turn the ankle down, with the toes pointed downward, you are *plantar flexing* the ankle.

Rotation describes movement around a longitudinal axis. When you turn your head from side to side, you are rotating your neck and changing the angle in relation to the trunk. Holding your hands up, as when under arrest, involves "external rotation" of the shoulder joint. When you walk along with your hands clasped behind your back, the shoulder joints are in "internal rotation." If you are sitting on the edge of an examining table with your legs dangling, and I pull your lower leg out to the side from the ankle, I am actually internally rotating your hip. If I pull it in and across your other leg, I am externally rotating your hip.

Then there are *pronation* and *supination*. If you are lying on your stomach, you are in the prone position. If you are lying on your back, you are supine. Pronation and supination also describe motions at the wrists and feet. The way I remember the distinction is: If you reach your hand out, palm up, in a begging or supplicating gesture, you have just "supinated" your wrist joint. The opposite, turning it over so that the palm faces downward, involves pronation.

With so many people running these days, you hear a lot more about pronation and supination of the feet than you used to. In fact, an entry in this book is devoted to problems of pronation and supination (see page 222). But briefly, supination of the foot means that the bottom surface of the foot is angled inward and up toward a "sole-up" position analagous to the "palm-up" position of a supinated wrist joint. It puts a lot of weight on the outside edge of the foot. Pronation is the opposite, with the weight shifting to the inner side of the foot.

It may be helpful to know the terms "proximal" and "distal." *Proximal* means "near to." For instance, if I talk about weakness in your proximal muscles, I am referring primarily to your shoulder and hip muscles, which are *close to* the trunk of your body. *Distal* means "far from," and so the muscles that move your wrists and ankles, which are farther away from the center of your body, are located "distally." *Peripheral* also means "farther away," but for some reason we don't talk about peripheral muscles. We do, however, refer to nerves that travel away from the spinal cord, and *out* to the arms and legs, as "peripheral nerves"—that is, peripheral to the central nervous system, the brain, and the spinal cord. When blood vessels that have traveled away from the heart and out toward the hands and feet no longer function effectively, we talk about "peripheral vascular disease."

BALANCE

The art of walking upright, however casually we may accept it, is in fact an incredible balancing act, one in which three major systems must function effectively in order to avoid sudden and dangerous disruptions. Loss of nervous system sensitivity, reduced blood flow to the brain, and muscle weakness can all disrupt the motor sequence and lead to a temporary loss of balance, resulting in a frightening and dangerous fall.

Such incidents should never be taken lightly, for they may have serious causes and consequences. So if you experience any sudden loss of balance—especially if you also lose consciousness—take the time to see a neurologist. Don't just attribute the problem to advancing years. Inner ear problems, heart irregularities, brain tumors, and prestroke attacks can all disrupt balance and consciousness, so pay attention to these possibly important warning signs.

Of course, the likelihood of such incidents increases as we grow older. By the seventh decade of life there is a reduction in the sensory feedback that informs you of your body's positions and actions. One way to compensate for this loss, a simple alternative of which you may not be aware, is to spread your feet and shorten your stride so that your gait approximates the gait you had as a very young child. Then, too, the interacting musculoskeletal and neurological systems may lose their sharpness as you grow older, and during the walking cycle this can lead to sudden loss of leg support and a fall. The gluteus medius muscle in your hip, for example, sustains most of the weight of your body when you step from one foot to the other. If it is weak, you may develop a waddling type of limp. If it gives way, you could stumble and fall.

Should you be faced with problems of balance and stability, problems that may range from modest to extremely serious, what do you do? First you go to the doctor and have them checked out. If your physician doesn't find any specific or correctable problem, there are two basic approaches to consider.

The first is to make the most of the physical resources you retain, which may be considerably more effective than you realize, especially if you work to improve them. Let me assure you, we all lose capacity as we grow older. But if we work to exploit the resources we have, we can maintain high levels of performance well into our later years. Thirty years ago, few people in their sixties and seventies played tennis; today, there are thousands and thousands of players in these age groups.

The second approach is to use a cane or other form of support. Such devices can be enormously helpful in getting you up and around, and of course walking can be crucial not only in maintaining the tone of your muscles and general physical condition but in permitting you to pursue your normal daily activities and routines.

To provide adequate assistance as a balance point, a cane must be cut so that when you are standing and the cane tip is on the floor, your elbow is bent at a 25- to 30-degree angle. This makes it possible for you to fully extend your arm when you step forward and lift your body, so that your arm and the cane form a single, nearly straight supportive unit. The end of your cane should have a rubber tip to keep it from slipping.

When a cane is used as a balance point, and not for a specific leg or hip problem, you should carry it in the hand that is most comfortable for you. When the cane hits the ground, it should be about six inches in front and to the side of your foot. If, however, you are using a cane to help support a painful leg or hip, then you must use it on the side opposite to your disability. This is important to keep your center of gravity beneath you, at a point between your injured leg and the cane. If you use the cane on the same side as your disability, then your center of gravity will shift to a point between your injured leg and the cane, and your already painful leg, which you are trying to protect, will have to bear even more weight. The cane and the foot on the painful side should hit the ground at the same time. You should really feel the cane hitting the ground as you transfer weight to it from the injured side.

Exercises for balance problems should be performed under very careful supervision, which can often best be provided by a physiatrist in a medical center or in a rehabilitation facility. I will not discuss specific exercises here, but there are many muscle-strengthening and balance-enhancing techniques that can help.

There is one consequence of losing your balance and falling that I want to be sure you know about. It is called a subdural hematoma. This is an accumulation of blood between the dura, or hard outer covering of the brain, and the brain itself and is caused by ruptured blood vessels. As we get older our blood vessels become more fragile and more vulnerable to rupture and leaking. A bump on the head against a cupboard door or a tree branch—or, of course, an actual fall—can set off this kind of bleeding. Since

you may not have any symptoms for several weeks, it is quite natural to forget or ignore that you hit your head in the first place. I know of a research project in which a subject was wired with a sensitive device and was found to have knocked his elbow against various objects over a hundred times a day without being aware of it! Anyway, a subdural hematoma can cause severe disabilities, and as a diagnosis it can easily be missed. The symptoms tend to come and go. You may be confused one day, or have some balance or speech difficulties, and then seem quite fine the next day. If you or your friends or family members notice something like this, be sure to see a neurologist or neurosurgeon right away. With the advent of CAT scans for the brain, a diagnosis can be made readily. A neurosurgeon can remove the blood and relieve the pressure on your brain by drilling some holes in your skull. I know this sounds gruesome, but it is really a simple procedure, and the benefits are immeasurable.

BICEPS TEAR

Perhaps the most popularly appreciated of all muscles, the biceps fills the upper arm with two bundles of fibers, known as the long head (upper bundle) and the short head (lower bundle), according to the differing lengths of the tendons that attach the fibers to the shoulder bones. The biceps bends the elbow and rotates the forearm to the palm-upward, or supinated position, and with regular exercise, and/or weight lifting, it can be built to impressive proportions. People who frequently use wrenches or screwdrivers, such as airplane mechanics, may have large bulging biceps muscles even though they don't lift weights.

Occasionally, when your elbow is bent and you are lifting a weight greater than what your muscles can tolerate, you may feel a sudden pop in your upper arm. If this happens you have probably torn a portion of your biceps. Though not a common injury, it does occur, especially in men and women in their fifties and sixties involved in heavy lifting, either at work or during recreation. Usually in these cases, the overloaded muscle fibers tear at the long head of the biceps where they intersect with the tendon. As a result, a bulge of loosened muscle fibers appears in the middle of the biceps along with a slight depression near the top of the upper arm.

This is not a serious injury. A typical biceps rupture results in only a 20 percent loss of total flexion and rotation strength, a loss that cannot be noticed in the performance of usual daily activities. However, it is important to apply ice and do some gentle flexion and extending of the elbow during the first week to ten days to reduce the pain and keep the muscles from tightening up as they heal over with fibrous tissue.

The torn fibers will never be as strong as they were before the rupture, but those fibers that are intact can be made stronger with regular exercise. Even if you are a competitive athlete, I would recommend that you build up these fibers rather than undergo surgical reattachment, which should only be done for cosmetic reasons.

EXERCISE 1

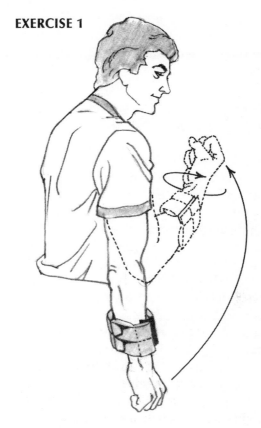

EXERCISE 1

After two weeks' healing, start exercising to rebuild your biceps. Start with a 1-pound weight around your wrist, your arm at your side, and your palm down. Slowly turn your fist upward and flex your elbow as far as you can. Do this 8 times. Remember to breathe regularly while exercising, and to relax between repetitions. When you can do 15 repetitions without straining, increase weight by a pound, drop back to 8 repetitions. Proceed in the same manner until you can do 15 repetitions with 10 pounds.

BREAST CANCER

Medical science has made enormous strides in detecting, destroying, and removing cancerous cells. Yet the problem of cancer remains one of the most troubling in all of medicine, and in no area is the battle more complex and emotional than in the treatment of breast cancer. I frequently work with breast cancer patients, and I am aware of the sensitive and sometimes difficult decisions they have to make.

More than 110,000 women in the United States develop cancer of the breast each year, making it the most common type of cancer among women (men do develop it occasionally). For slightly less than half of them, the choice of which operation to have is a relatively simple one. If cancerous cells, when detected, have spread into neighboring lymph glands, a modified radical mastectomy, or surgical removal of the whole breast, may be called for, along with removal of some muscle tissue and lymph nodes. This may be followed by radiation treatments and chemotherapy.

The remaining 50 percent of breast cancer patients belong to a group in which early detection establishes, to a high degree of certainty, that the focus of the cancer cells is limited to one area, and has not spread to the lymph nodes. A patient in this group has two choices: either the modified radical mastectomy or a lumpectomy, the surgical removal of the lump or mass alone, without removing the whole breast, followed by radiation.

Whichever procedure is chosen, a structured exercise program afterward can be enormously beneficial.

The exercises that are presented at the end of this section may be done after a mastectomy, or after a lumpectomy and while you are receiving radiation. These exercises were developed by the Rehabilitation Service at the Memorial Sloan-Kettering Cancer Center.

Even the modest surgery involved in a lumpectomy can keep you from moving your shoulder for fear of pain or of loosening stitches. Radiation, although it may produce no immediate unfavorable reactions, may lead to some tightening up of the tissues that have been treated. In a modified radical mastectomy with the breast, lymph nodes, and pectoralis minor muscle removed, a fairly major change in the chest and shoulder area takes place that will affect the surrounding muscles and how you use them. They must therefore be loosened and strengthened to help you use your arm and shoulder in a normal fashion.

The lymph tract drains the lymph fluid out of the forearm and upper arm into the venous system. If the lymph nodes under the arm are removed, these tracts are interrupted and the lymph fluid backs up and causes edema, a swelling in the arm and hand. The exercises outlined below and the application of a gradient compression sleeve can help reduce this edema.

If the condition reappears—as it may from changes in the remaining lymph nodes or from a mild infection (a so-called cellulitis)—it may be necessary to elevate the arm in a special sling at night while you sleep and then, when the swelling has subsided, to use an elastic gradient pressure stocking to keep fluid from gathering in the forearm. You should also avoid wearing a bra with a tight shoulder strap, one that cuts into the shoulder, as well as tight bracelets, watch bands, and sleeves. About 40 percent of lymph is carried through the subdermal or skin lymph complex, which is not affected by surgery, so you don't want to wear anything that will impair the flow of lymph through this part of the system.

It is also important to remember that lymph glands and ducts are part of your primary line of defense against invading organisms, and once they have been cut out you must guard against infection at all times. Threats to consider include everything from cuts, scratches, and vaccinations, to burns, sunburn, even detergents that may irritate your hands. Your arm is vulnerable; you must guard it vigilantly. When you feel increased tightness in your arm, or you notice that the arm is getting bigger, you have already accumulated about 1,000 cc of fluid. You should consult a physiatrist or your breast surgeon to determine the cause of the edema and what to do about it. We suggest that you begin the following exercises the day after surgery, but you should check with your doctor before doing so.

EXERCISE 1

This exercise is designed to stretch and rotate your shoulder. Sit in a straight-backed chair with your feet flat on the floor and your hands at your sides. Raise your arms to shoulder height and extend them straight out to the side. With both arms up, move the arm on the side that has been treated up and to the rear, as if you were doing the backstroke. Make a counterclockwise circle for 5 repetitions, relax, and do again 3 to 5 times.

EXERCISE 1

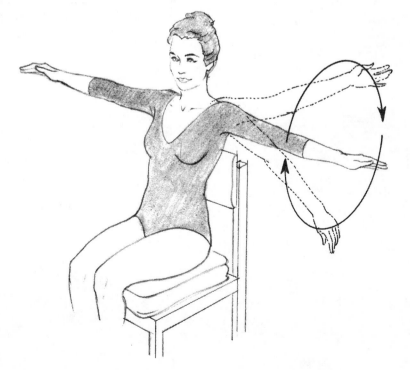

EXERCISE 2

This exercise will help loosen and stretch the muscles in the area of your treatment. Sit in a straight-backed chair with your feet flat on the floor and your hands at your sides. Clasp your hands in front of your stomach; slowly raise your hands up over your head and down onto the back of your neck. Bring your elbows out to the side as far as you can without pain. In this position, slowly rotate the upper part of your body away from the treatment side, hold for 5 seconds (count to 6), then return to the starting position. Gradually build up to 5 repetitions. This exercise stretches the pectoralis muscles and latissimus dorsi muscles.

EXERCISE 2

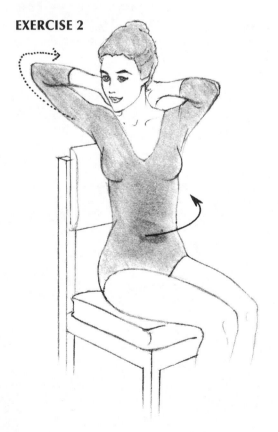

EXERCISE 3

This two-part stretching exercise will help loosen muscles in both your back and chest. Do not force your movement or strain to complete the exercise. Stand upright with your feet about 6 inches apart, arms straight in front of your body. Holding a rolled towel in your hands slowly bring it up and over your head, behind your neck, and toward your upper back as far as you can without pain. Do not arch your back. Do not strain. Hold your maximum comfortable position for 5 seconds (count to 6), then return to the starting position. The second part of this exercise is the same as the first except you're holding the towel behind you. In this position, gently raise your arms up and away from your body as far as you can without straining. Hold your maximum comfortable position for 5 seconds (count to 6), then relax. Begin with a single repetition of both exercises and build gradually to 5.

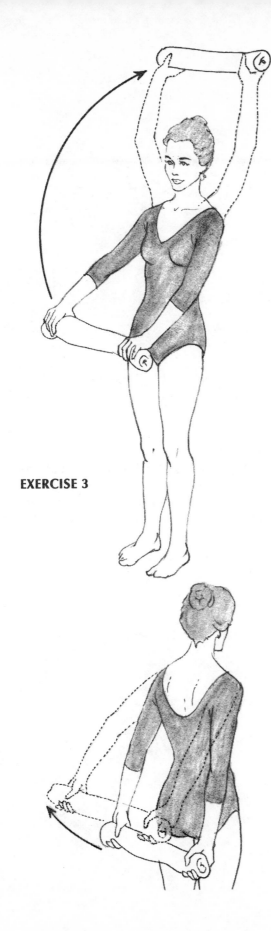

EXERCISE 4

This exercise will help loosen muscles in your shoulder and upper back. Sit on a flat stool with your back straight, arms at your sides, and your feet flat on the floor. Reach behind your back with your treatment arm and gradually attempt to touch the bottom of the opposite shoulder blade, going only as far as is comfortable. Hold for 5 seconds (count to 6), then relax and let your arms rest normally at your side. Start with one repetition and build gradually to 10.

EXERCISE 4

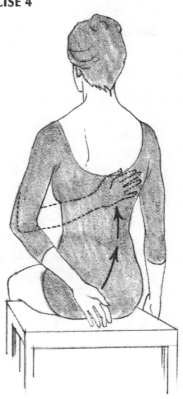

EXERCISE 3

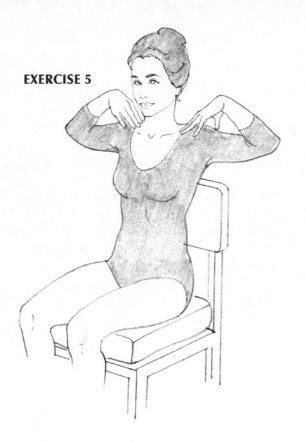

EXERCISE 5

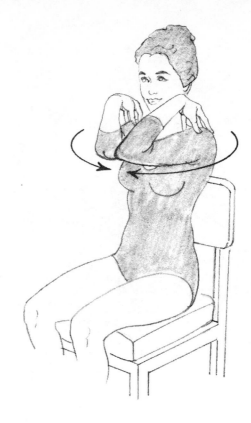

EXERCISE 5

This exercise will stretch your back and shoulder muscles. Sit in a straight-backed chair with your feet flat on the floor and your hands at your sides. Place the fingers of your right hand on your right shoulder and the fingers of your left hand on your left shoulder. Now, slowly try to bring your elbows together at shoulder height and touch in front of your chin. Hold this position for 5 seconds (count to 6), then return to the starting position and relax. Start with a single repetition and work up to 5. Exhale as you bring your arms forward.

EXERCISE 6

This is a range-of-motion exercise to test your progress. From about a foot away, stand and face a wall, place the hand of the

unaffected arm as high on the wall as you can and make a mark at that level. If you have undergone a bilateral mastectomy, or had decreased range before surgery (be-

EXERCISE 6

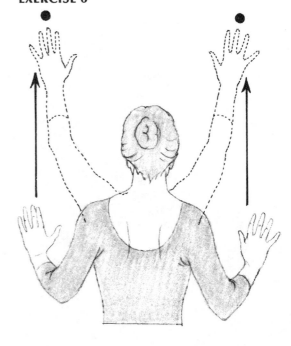

cause of arthritis, for example), your goal will be to attain your presurgical ranges of motion. You begin by placing both hands on the wall at shoulder height. Slowly walk both hands up the wall until you begin to feel tightness or pain on the mastectomy side. Make a mark on the wall at this spot, then hold it for 5 seconds (count to 6) before walking your hands back down to the starting position. Repeat 5 times. Each day you will find that you are able to reach a bit higher, and finally you will be able to touch the mark of your unaffected arm.

EXERCISE 7

This is known as the pendulum, or limp-swing, exercise. Stand behind a straight-backed chair that has a low back. Place the hand of the unaffected arm on the back of the chair. Let your treated arm hang down loosely until your elbow, wrist, and hand are all fully extended. Gently swing your arm from left to right, making sure your shoulder and not your arm supplies the movement. Keep the elbow stiff. When your arm is fully relaxed, begin to swing it in small circles as shown in the illustration below. Gradually increase the size of the circles, then reverse their direction. There is no set number of swings; stop the exercise when your arms feel loose and relaxed. About one week after you leave the hospital, discontinue this exercise to avoid fluid accumulation in the arm.

EXERCISE 7

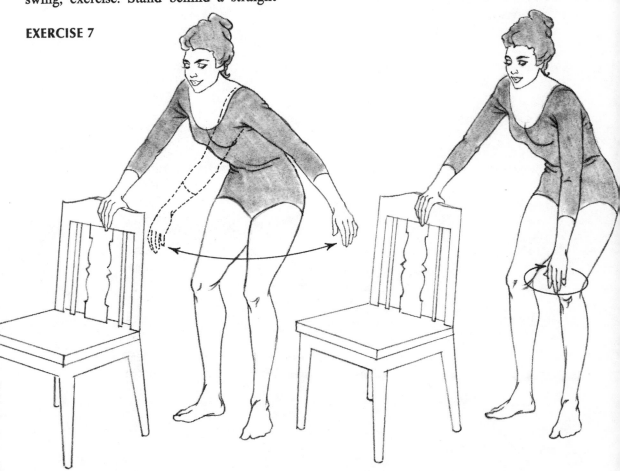

EXERCISE 8

This exercise is designed to loosen damaged tissues. Sit in a comfortable straight-backed chair with your feet flat on the floor and clasp your hands in your lap. With fingers interlaced, slowly raise your hands toward your face. If you feel pain or tightness, stop and breathe deeply until the discomfort eases. Continue lifting your hands until you reach the top of your head. If you are free of pain in this position, move your clasped hands down behind your neck, keeping your head upright. When you are comfortable in this position, spread your elbows apart and hold for 5 seconds (count to 6). If pulling or discomfort occurs, return to starting position. Do this exercise 3 times.

EXERCISE 8

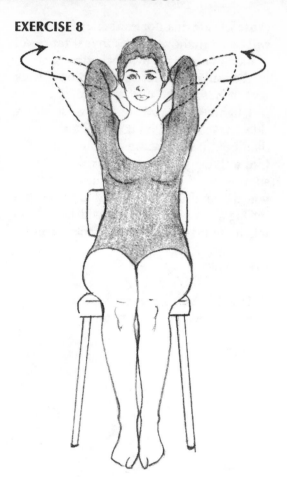

EXERCISE 9

EXERCISE 9

This exercise is designed to increase range of motion in your affected arm by stretching the shoulder muscles. To do it, you need a straight-backed chair, a pulley or hook firmly attached high up a wall, and a 3- to 4-foot section of soft rope with handles at both ends. Sit in the chair (directly under the pulley or hook) with your feet flat on the floor and your back to the wall. Grasp the rope as high up as possible with the hand of your uninjured arm, then grasp the other handle with your treated hand and begin to pull the rope down until you feel pain in the treated side. Stop and relax for a few moments in this position, breathe deeply. If deep breathing relieves the pain, continue slowly pulling your treated arm upward. Stop again when it hurts, breathe deeply once more, and slowly return to the point where you first felt pain to repeat as before. Your goal: to raise both arms to the same height.

If you have had a bilateral mastectomy, use chair, rope handles, and hook as above, but inch up your less painful arm until you feel pain. Stop, let your arms relax in this position, and breathe deeply. Once the pain has eased, continue raising the arm in this manner as long as breathing eases the pain. Repeat the exercise, using your other arm to raise the arm with which you first began the exercise. Your goal should be to build up both arms so that you can reach as high above your head as you could before surgery.

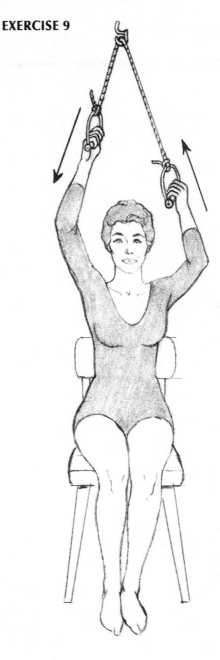

EXERCISE 10

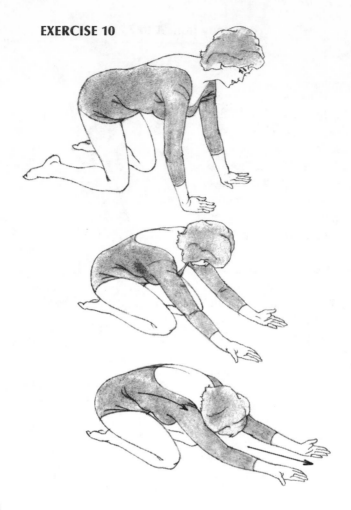

EXERCISE 10

This is for stretching your pectoralis muscles. Get down on your hands and knees with hands under your shoulders, elbows straight, and palms flat on the floor. Leaning back on your haunches, turn your palms upward. Holding that position, stretch your arms forward as far as possible. You should feel a pull in the front of your chest and below the shoulders. Hold this stretched position for 5 seconds (count to 6), then return to the original position. Repeat the exercise 5 times.

BURSITIS

The body's joints are dotted with bursae, soft sacs that produce lubricating synovial fluid and help provide a cushioning effect between tendons and bones. There are more than a dozen bursae in the knee, for example, while others pad the elbow and heel, or smooth the operations of the shoulder and hip, helping tendon glide over bone. In all, about 150 of these protective "oil cans" serve the body. There is no firm figure, however, because new bursae can actually be created by friction and irritation.

Bursae can become painful and inflamed when overused, bruised, or subjected to prolonged external pressure. They tend to overreact by swelling up and secreting more synovial fluid than they would normally. Housemaid's knee, for example, is a form of bursitis that develops from spending long periods of time scrubbing floors in a kneeling position. In the hospital we sometimes see patients with a trochanteric bursitis in the hip area; the trochanter is part of the large bone that fits into the hip joint and the problem develops when patients lie on their sides for prolonged periods. The shoulder, elbow, and heel are similarly susceptible.

For any type of bursitis, cold is the best treatment. Applying an ice pack for twenty minutes at a time, two or even three times a day for several days, can damp down a throbbing bursa and return it to its normal functions. Aspirin will usually help the pain. In some cases, it may be necessary to give a cortisone injection directly into the bursa to decrease the inflammation. A group of medicines called nonsteroidal anti-inflammatory agents can be helpful. The one thing you must not do is use heat to ease the pain and swelling. Heat will only make the fluid inside a bursa expand and the bursa to produce additional fluid.

In extremely rare instances, simple surgery may be performed to remove an offending bursa. I myself have never found it necessary to recommend surgery for bursitis, and although I have seen people re-ceive relief from removal of a bursa, sooner or later a new one forms and acts up at the same site. Bursae have a tendency to do this.

Whenever you have pain in a joint, you will favor it and try not to move it too much. This can result, for example, in a frozen shoulder and loss of strength in the shoulder muscles. As soon as the acute pain of a bursitis subsides—with the help of a cortisone injection or cold application—you should start moving your joint gently so it will not lose its range of motion. It is harder to get this function back than to strengthen muscles that have been allowed to weaken. If you are able to maintain the normal range of motion of the joint afflicted with bursitis, you have achieved a great deal. The bursitis may subside by itself, but I don't believe in counting on this. Besides, the cortisone-plus-exercise treatment we recommend carries hardly any risk.

CARDIAC REHABILITATION

Here is one aspect of rehabilitation medicine that has established a secure and important position in the management of patients following heart attacks or coronary bypass surgery. Cardiac rehabilitation is based on the principle that the undamaged heart muscle can be trained to perform efficiently. This principle is basically the same as it is for other muscles in the body: You can't increase the number of muscle fibers, but you can increase the efficiency of those you have.

A cardiac rehabilitation program is administered according to the MET principle. Each activity has a certain energy requirement, and this requirement can be expressed in METs, or metabolic equivalents. For example, sitting in a chair has a MET value of one. Bending forward and making a bed requires three METs; raking leaves, five METs; and jogging eight METs. This is highly convenient, for it lets you see how much energy expenditure a patient can tolerate by using a treadmill under careful cardiac monitoring and translating the observed tolerance into a capacity for other activities. Not only does this enable the physician to advise the patient about the kind of activities that can safely be engaged in, it can also guide both through a structured program of gradually increasing levels of exertion. A cardiac rehabilitation program is similar in principle to training programs for healthy people who wish to increase their aerobic capacity.

A lot of people who have had heart attacks or have undergone a coronary bypass procedure are anxious to return to their former level of activity, or even to improve it. For these I strongly recommend participating in a cardiac rehabilitation program under the supervision of a cardiologist, or a physiatrist with a particular interest in this area, working with specially trained physical therapists. A good program of this kind can enhance the probability of tolerating increased levels of activity well, including, in many cases, athletic activity. At New York Hospital we have a special cardiac rehabilitation program for all inpatients who have undergone coronary bypass or valve replacement procedures. It is initiated before they go home; and thereafter, even following full recovery, the patients are guided through an outpatient program at various cardiac rehabilitation centers, or at private offices run by physicians with experience in cardiac rehabilitation.

CARPAL TUNNEL SYNDROME

The anatomical design of the body narrows at certain points, such as the neck and wrist, in such a way that substantial amounts of bone, muscle, tendon, and nerve have to be packed into a relatively tight space. If one of these components acts up, a painful problem can result.

This is what happens in carpal tunnel syndrome, a wrist problem that occurs more frequently, especially among women approaching middle age, than its exotic-sounding name might indicate. The term is actually very apt, for the carpal tunnel is formed by the wrist bones (known as the carpals) and the transverse ligament. It is situated on the palm side of the wrist joint. The carpal bones are held in place by this ligament that runs across the base of the palm like the strap of a watch. Through this short tunnel pass the tendons that travel down the wrist and move the fingers. The median nerve, which supplies the muscles that allow you to move your thumb and make a fist, also shares space in this cramped passageway. If your finger-operating tendons become irritated because of overuse, they may swell and press on this nerve. Painting, digging ditches, playing racquetball, working on an assembly line, playing the piano—any of these can create reactions inside the carpal tunnel that put pressure on the nerve, as can the retention of fluid in the body.

The symptoms of such compression may be slight at first, a tingling feeling in the thumb and second and third fingers, sometimes part of the fourth finger (but never the fifth). You may also feel some numbness in the fingers. Discomfort may become worse at night while you sleep, even to the point of waking you up. If this occurs, you can ease the tingling and numbness by shaking your hand or hanging it over the edge of the bed, which is why many people at first think the problem is circulatory rather than nerve-related. But during sleep you may be inadvertantly putting your hand in a position that increases the pressure on the nerve. Shaking your hand may give you some relief simply because you are holding the hand in a more advantageous position, and not because you are increasing the blood flow to the fingers. In any event, it is important to have this condition evaluated before the muscles that move the thumb weaken.

If you were to arrive at my office complaining of numbness and tingling in your hand, I would bend your wrist back so that your palm is almost perpendicular to your forearm, and hold it there for a few seconds to see if the position aggravates the numbness and tingling. I might also press my thumbs directly on the ligaments that form the tunnel, or tap them with a reflex hammer. A sudden flash of tingling in the thumb and index finger would be a positive Tinel's sign, indicating compression of the median nerve. To confirm the diagnosis, I would use an electrodiagnostic test that would show the extent of nerve damage. This is called a nerve conduction study and measures the nerve's ability to carry an electrical impulse over a certain distance within a given time span. If carpal tunnel syndrome is present, the time it takes for a stimulus to travel from the wrist to the muscles of the thumb is prolonged. I'd also want to make sure that the problem wasn't coming from higher up along the course of the median nerve, even as far up as the neck.

I would also use a procedure called "electromyography" to measure the electrical activity of the muscles controlled by the median nerve. This involves placing a very fine needle electrode into the muscle itself.

Treatment really depends on the extent of nerve compression and muscle weakness. In some cases, diuretics (which drain water from the body) can help. I usually recommend the patient to one of our occupational therapists who would make a static wrist splint, which one wears at night. (It is called static because it does not allow movement, and holds the wrist in one position.) You would wear the splint at night to prevent your hand from drifting into positions that would press on the nerve. You could buy such a splint in a surgical supply store, but I strongly recommend that you have one custom-made. It is usually much more comfortable, and comfort is vital, since you may have to wear the splint for three or four weeks, until the numbness or pain subsides. Proper fit is also very important; if the splint is too tight it may cause more swelling and aggravate the problem; if the splint is too loose, it doesn't give you any protection at all.

Should the splint not bring you any relief, or if your case was already quite advanced by the time it was diagnosed, you would probably have to undergo a simple surgical procedure. The surgeon increases the room for your median nerve by cutting through the tough ligament at the base of the tunnel. The operation normally requires only a brief hospital stay and leaves just the slightest of scars on the inside of the wrist.

In the event you do undergo surgery, you may also need some rehabilitation afterward. Sometimes the muscles of the thumb weaken or the wrist stiffens after surgery. A short program of range of motion and strengthening exercises is often very helpful. A skilled occupational therapist can instruct you in these exercises and maneuvers. You can do them by yourself at home, with rechecks every second week for the next four to six weeks.

Some physicians may recommend oral anti-inflammatory medication, or a steroid injection into the carpal tunnel. I am not in favor of either approach. You have to take a great deal of medication by mouth for it to enter your system and affect a local condition. As for the steroid injection: I consider myself a pretty good marksman when it comes to injections, but I would not dare to inject anywhere near the median nerve; I might just hit it and cause more pain!

CARTILAGE

The ends of the bones that form our joints are covered with a smooth, white, glistening material known as cartilage. Con-

stantly lubricated by synovial fluid, cartilage gives ball-bearing slickness to the insides of joints and helps them move easily and rapidly in response to the contractions of the muscles.

The passage of time gradually wears down the cartilage in our joints, making movement less smooth. Excessive wear can lead to the formation of rough, uneven, patches and cause stiffness and pain in the joint. Menisci (meniscus in the singular), two circular pieces of cartilage in the knee, perform a kind of shock-absorbing function. Severe blows to the knee, or pivoting over the knee with the foot caught, or falling downhill with one ski caught in soft snow, can loosen and even tear these pads and cause extreme pain. In recent years, arthroscopic surgical techniques—in which tiny scissors are inserted into the joint along with a light source and a special lens—have made it possible to remove small, loosened sections of cartilage. This type of microsurgery avoids the debilitating effects of a full-scale operation and can return athletes to training in a matter of weeks. In many cases, however, a conservative, exercise-oriented approach is sufficient to produce results, especially on a long-term basis, that are just as good and don't require cutting into the joint.

If it looks as if you have a torn meniscus, I would advise the following: First, get some crutches so you can avoid putting weight on the side of the painful knee. Then go somewhere where you can rest and give yourself ice treatments, keeping the knee partially bent. Put ice on it every hour for twenty minutes at a time. When the swelling has subsided somewhat, try to contract your quadriceps muscle carefully by extending your knee and holding it for five seconds, then relaxing it. In many instances, the acute pain will subside to such a level that you can extend your knee fully.

If you are not able to do this, I would ask a physical therapist to apply some electrical stimulation to the area. This would help the quadriceps muscle contract, mobilize the fluid, and reduce the swelling. It may take two to three weeks for the pain and swelling to subside completely and for full motion of the joint to return. By that time your quadriceps muscle may have wasted substantially from disuse, and it will have to be strengthened. Your therapist will show you exercises for this and will practice walking with you, showing or reminding you how to use the heel-to-toe gait. You should gradually be able to return to your regular activities, but I would strongly advise the use of a knee brace with lateral enforcements if you start to participate in athletics again.

There are three situations where I would recommend surgery. The first is if you are a professional athlete and time is of the essence. The second is if you have frequent recurrent problems with the menisci in your knee. And the third is if you continue to have severe pain and find that the range of motion in your knee does not improve after ten to twelve days.

I've heard two conflicting arguments about surgical intervention for meniscus problems in the knee. One is that without an operation the chances of developing osteoarthritis in the knee later are increased. The other is that *with* the operation you can develop osteoarthritis of the knee later (now surgeons try to remove as little as possible from the meniscus). Either way,

the jury is still out on the long-term effects of arthroscopic knee surgery. The big advantage of this procedure is that the knee joint does not have to be opened. Still, I would encourage you to consider everything very carefully before making a decision. And whatever your decision, don't go back to your athletic activities before you have rehabilitated your quadriceps.

CHARLEY HORSE

The term "charley horse" may have originated as a description of a lame horse by the name of Charley, or possibly the owner's name was Charley. All we know for sure is that nowadays the phrase most often designates the pain resulting from overexertion of a muscle. Today it is also known as Delayed Onset Muscle Tension (DOMT).

This means that the muscle has been worked to such an extent that it is unable to rid itself of accumulated waste products, such as lactic acid and carbon dioxide. It's possible, too, that some tiny muscle tears have taken place and caused a small amount of bleeding. Overloading an unprepared muscle can cause pain or soreness the following day, or even two days later, and this in turn can sometimes trigger muscle spasms.

In most cases, however, a charley horse refers simply to a tight and very sore muscle, not one that is in spasm. You can ease the discomfort of a charley horse by applying hot packs for twenty minutes at a time, several times a day, or by taking frequent hot baths. Heat will help to dilate the small blood vessels and remove waste products through increased circulation (I prefer to reserve ice for those situations in which there is visible swelling and the muscle is really in spasm). The soreness should disappear gradually in four or five days, and during this time you should keep mildly active by walking or gently stretching the aching muscles.

CHIROPRACTIC

Many chiropractors are knowledgeable and skilled professionals capable of helping their patients. While they do not undergo as many years of rigorous and comprehensive training as do medical doctors, they are well-versed in anatomy, particularly the anatomy of the musculoskeletal system. The backbone (no pun intended!) of their treatment approach is spinal manipulation, a procedure in which quick, deft pressure is brought to the spinal area in an attempt to restore it to its proper alignment, thereby relieving various ailments and afflictions, including back pain.

So far so good. What I have trouble with is the following. A chiropractor usually takes an X-ray of your spine using a special grid with a pattern of intersecting perpendicular lines. These lines are then used to impress on you how poor the alignment of your spine is and how ripe it is for some chiropractic adjustment. It is true that X-rays can be helpful in showing an abnormal side-to-side spinal curvature called scoliosis, but it is very rare to find a spine that is absolutely straight as an arrow. I am familiar with a study of 1,000 healthy young men in which only twenty-eight more or less straight spines were found on X-ray. And this is not surprising; after the age of four or so the configuration of our spines is largely determined by our needs and activities. Those activities may vary from minimal to very active and athletic, and the muscles on one side of the body may be used and developed more than those on the other. Whatever the degree of activity, no two spines will look completely alike, and very few will be held in place by perfectly balanced forces. In other words, an imperfect alignment is actually quite normal and therefore should not be used as a premise for manipulation of the back.

What exactly do chiropractors achieve with their techniques? We all know people who have felt better after a chiropractic treatment. Certainly chiropractors can loosen up the tight muscles that may be causing back pain, but not as a result of adjusting the spine, as they often claim. The lower spine is held together by ligaments, tendons, joints, and muscles that combine to exert powerful mechanical forces on the area. To overcome such forces with a swift movement of the hands would, in my opinion, be virtually impossible. The muscles might be loosened up somewhat, but that would be all. The X-ray might then show a better adjustment against the grid, but that would be because the slight pull of a tight muscle on one side of the spine has now been released and the spine accordingly appears straighter. Nothing, however, would have been done to change the fundamental interlocking structures of the spine.

Chiropractors may also be favored (as all good physicians are) by the placebo effect. I remember a patient who insisted that I perform an adjustment on him. When I demurred, he became quite upset and suggested that I was being unduly harsh and unfair. I decided it would be in his best interests for me to perform a maneuver rather than to deny him, and so I gently and harmlessly brought his right leg out to the side and his knee to his chest. Moments later, the patient leapt up happily, claiming that he had never experienced such skillful adjustment. All that I could possibly have done was relax a tight muscle, and I'm not even sure I did that!

One simple and important thing that most chiropractors do is examine and touch the human body. This is still an important part of any physical exam, despite all the testing we do and questions we ask. Complex tests don't always solve complex problems, but a good physical exam can. I remember a patient who came to me at the suggestion of a chiropractor. She had hurt her shoulder on the sharp edge of a crate, damaging the nerve that controlled the muscle that moved her shoulder blade. She had been seen by various specialists who had found nothing specifically wrong and had prescribed painkillers, which only relieved her pain temporarily. In desperation, she went to a chiropractor who looked at her carefully, examined both shoulders, compared them, and told her she had a winged scapula, or protruding shoulder blade, resulting from a damaged nerve. He advised her to call me. The chiropractor was right, and we were able to help.

Should you go to a chiropractor? Personally, I have never found myself in a position where it seemed advisable to send someone to a chiropractor—it's always

been the other way around. I suppose this is because I have so much confidence in the techniques that my field has to offer. These techniques are based on sound anatomical and physiological principles, and after years of using them and developing them I have seen that they provide long-term benefits for my patients that other approaches can't offer.

If you should go to a chiropractor, I would strongly urge you to avoid any sort of manipulation that involves the neck. This is an extremely delicate area containing a complex network of nerves and blood vessels. An abrupt, forceful manipulation there can lead to a number of problems including, tragically, stroke. It won't happen very often, but several cases have been reported in the literature, so I believe it's a chance you shouldn't take.

Is chiropractic worthwhile? It would be best, in my opinion, for the medical establishment to undertake a careful study of all chiropractic techniques, one designed to determine exactly what it is chiropractors can and cannot achieve. And then perhaps the positive aspects of chiropractic might be incorporated into standard patient care in the United States.

COLD AND HEAT TREATMENTS

Cold—applied in the form of ice, ice packs, or ethyl chloride spray—is one of the simplest and most effective weapons in the physiatrist's arsenal. Applications of cold may be used to treat everything from muscle spasms and tears to torn tendons and inflammation. Perhaps the most surprising aspect of the use of cold treatment is not its effectiveness, for that has been clearly established, but the reluctance with which some patients use it and some doctors prescribe it.

For a long time heat—in the form of hot baths, heating pads, or warm whirlpools—was the prevailing physical agent for soothing pain. Indeed, heat does feel very soothing, and it is just the thing to use if one has tight muscles. Thus, when I tell patients to prepare and apply ice, I often detect reluctance on their part, perhaps because cold is frequently associated with discomfort. Yet in certain instances, cold will actually provide superior physiological benefits.

With acute injuries, ice is much more effective in decreasing the pain and swelling. What it does is slow down the nerve's ability to conduct painful stimuli—a process called reflex vasoconstriction—thereby breaking into the viscious cycle of muscle spasm, pain, and muscle spasm. It also causes the blood vessels to constrict and retard the leakage of fluid into the surrounding tissues. This is followed by the opposite phenomenon of reflex vasodilation, which means that the blood vessels now dilate or expand spontaneously, allowing more blood to flow to the muscle in spasm. Since much of the pain of muscle spasm comes from a relatively low supply of blood (ischemia), this new supply, with the oxygen it carries, also helps to reduce the pain.

Heat, too, increases blood flow by dilating the blood vessels, and by helping to deliver oxygen and carry off waste products. Heat is therefore good for sore or overused muscles. It is, however, not as effective as ice for muscle *spasm*. Apparently, the combination of vasoconstriction followed by vasodilation that ice provides is much more powerful.

Heat can also help you to unwind and relax. A warm tub or whirlpool bath can be a great and soothing treat for your whole body after a long day of hiking or golf.

Heat should never be used during the acute phase of any muscle, tendon, or ligament injury because it will promote the leakage of fluid from the blood vessels and lead to increased rather than decreased swelling. Nor should heat be used for an acute bursitis, where it will cause expansion of the fluid inside a bursal sac.

There are three basic methods of delivering cold to the surface of the skin and the injured tissues below it. Ethyl chloride spray, a liquid that can be squirted on, is probably the easiest to use (which is why it is often seen in the hands of trainers at athletic events). Cold packs, which are sold in drugstores, can be chilled in the freezer, and the gel inside will stay cold for a long time. But in the opinion of many experts, nothing beats ice itself. There are a number of ways to apply it. Plastic bags filled with ice chips are good, but a sheet or thin towel should be used to protect the skin against frostbite. You can also fill several paper cups with water, freeze them, then use them for an "ice massage" or direct application of ice onto the skin over a painful or swollen area.

If you wish to try the latter technique, fill several paper cups with water and put them in the freezer. When it comes time to massage a painful area, tear the paper away from the sides of the cup, exposing the ice but leaving the bottom paper portion for you to hold. Slowly massage the area of injury with short overlapping strokes. Be sure to keep the ice moving, otherwise you may slightly freeze and injure surface tissues.

Ice must always be used with care. In whatever form, it should be applied for fifteen to twenty minutes, but not longer. After that time it will have no beneficial physiological effect. Actually, the greatest benefit from ice accrues after twelve to fourteen minutes, but I suggest that you apply it for twenty minutes to make sure that you achieve maximum cooling beneath the surface of the skin. In extreme cases of muscle spasm, you may want to ice an area once every hour or so. When using ice in a pack or bag, be sure to cover the bag with a light cloth or towel to protect the skin.

The forms of heat that we are most familiar with are "superficial"—that is, the warmth does not penetrate very far into the body's tissues. In most rehabilitation departments you will find that hydrocollator packs are commonly used. They can be easily heated up in hot water, and the gel inside will hold the heat for a long time. There is nothing wrong with a hot water bottle or a hot moist terry cloth towel, but both will cool off before the heat can exert maximum effect (before the twenty minutes are up). When you use a hydrocollator pack, by the way, you should place a moist towel between the pack and the skin. This not only helps to protect the skin, it also transfers the heat *to* the skin.

In order for heat to penetrate more deeply into the body—say, all the way into the hip joint—it is necessary to use more sophisticated methods. You may have heard of shortwave and microwave diathermy machines, which aim their electromagnetic waves at the area to be treated. We don't use them because it is difficult to control the temperature effects in the body. Ultrasound, however, is a form of deep heat that we use very frequently and feel comfortable with.

COLLISION SPORTS

Not long ago I was invited to speak at a football dinner at an elegant New York club. Forty or so famous older players were there, and during the course of the evening each was asked to stand, introduce himself, and recall a play or game in which he had helped make gridiron history. Sometime after that dinner, one of the players, who was suffering from tennis elbow problems, came to see me as a patient. In the course of his treatment he asked me what had impressed me most about the dinner. I had to tell him the truth. I was struck by the fact that few of the players were able to stand up without holding onto their chairs and that many walked with some form of limp.

This is the downside of sports injuries, especially as we see them at New York Hospital. It is a side far removed from the cheers of the college crowd or the money and prestige of the professional game. Despite all the protective devices in use (and, in certain unfortunate cases, because of them) impact sports cause injury. Sports injuries should not be taken lightly. They can haunt you in later life. The truth is that collision injuries (and not necessarily fractures) can, like slow-fused time bombs, smolder for a decade or two and then cause very real and painful problems.

The rate of injury is still too high in football at all levels of the game. And, of course, you can get hurt by crashing into your opponents in hockey, soccer, and basketball, too. Rugby is also a case in point. I recall one patient, a dashing Australian who had suffered rugby injuries in his youth, who summed up the problem this way: "One thing I wish I had told my son is this: Don't play rugby. I'm a pretty good tennis player, but I can't play anymore because I had my knees banged up so badly. I'm healthy and feel I could keep on playing forever, but my knees won't let me."

What actually happens in the case of a delayed-reaction disability? When you cut yourself, you grow new skin to replace the old, but when your bones are traumatized over and over in the same spot, they respond in a slightly different manner: They grow new bone *over* the impact area. Eventually, this new, roughened layer may be substantial enough to press on a nerve (if your vertebrae are involved) or to make the operation of a joint painful (if your knee or shoulder have been knocked around). The initial injury doesn't have to be that damaging for this to happen. Often the team doctor may take an X-ray, see that nothing is broken, and send you back to play in the next game. This is perfectly normal. Unfortunately, you'll probably receive more blows in the same spot in the next game, some of them delivered in sledgehammer fashion by unbreakable steel and plastic helmets, and if enough land, the bone changing process will begin.

While this is a common scenario, I don't mean to suggest that football or hockey or soccer are bad games. They aren't; they are important in the growth and development of young people in this country, and we all need our heroes to root for. What I am suggesting is that many players—high school, college, and professional—are not aware that repeated blows to the neck, back, and knee can trigger the formation of bony spurs or other changes that may make their lives less enjoyable two decades later. I once discussed this problem with a trial lawyer, a man who had suffered neck injuries playing football in college. He suggested that if professional players fully understood the implications of their traumatic injuries, they might give more consideration to other career choices.

If you are a player or the parent of a player, what can you do? The solution is relatively simple, though perhaps not easily put into action. The time to protect yourself is when you are first injured, and this means letting the damage heal properly; resting and protecting the area for *at least two weeks*. It also usually means sitting out at least two games. Few players are prepared to do this, for when you are part of a team you are supposed to help your team, despite pain and injury. Please try to remember that you can help your team more in the short run, and yourself in the long run, if you allow enough time for the body to repair itself right after an injury.

This is a country of team sports, nearly all of them collision sports, and I am not against them. I just think that children and their parents should be aware of the risks and that everyone should engage in at least one noncollision sport that they really enjoy and can play all their lives.

Equipment changes and innovations have done a great deal to reduce the frequency of certain football injuries, but two pieces of equipment—helmets and face masks—can sometimes hurt as much as they help. Years ago, helmets were made of leather and weighed about a pound and a half. Such helmets didn't offer adequate protection (and perhaps more significant in the modern era of TV sports, they didn't take paint, varnish, and decals the way plastic helmets do). Today's four-pound plastic helmet with a one-pound steel face mask bolted to it provides excellent protection for the skull and face, including the nose and teeth. However, when that same four-pound helmet is driven into the back or ribs of another player, it becomes a dangerous weapon. And though rule changes have attempted to block such battering ram tactics, they don't always succeed. The face mask, looming like a cage in front of the face, suffers from another kind of duplicity. It offers excellent protection, but it can also transmit dangerous stresses to the spine if it is driven downward by the wearer, or tipped up and back by an opponent in the heat of battle. Since today's tight-fitting helmets don't slip, they dispatch external pounding and twisting directly to the head and neck. And indeed, while there are few broken noses these days, the rate of neck injuries has if anything increased.

Much has been done to improve equipment and cut down on the chances of injury, but one factor has not been adequately taken into consideration. Our youngsters are much taller and heavier than they were in the past, so the impact on collision is much greater than it used to be. The present protective equipment, though much improved, may still require further changes. There may also have to be more rule changes that take the increased height and weight of our young men into consideration.

CORTISONE INJECTIONS

Cortisone, cortisol, and corticosterone are three closely related substances that are naturally present in the human body. They are produced by two small almond-shaped organs, the adrenal glands, which are perched on top of the kidneys. They are involved in a wide variety of physiological activities, such as glucose production by the liver and the metabolism of fatty substances.

Synthetic cortisone and its relatives are also used for medical purposes, usually to help fight inflammatory reactions. They can be given orally or by injection. For the kind of musculoskeletal problems we talk about in this book, cortisone injections are definitely preferable because they can be aimed directly at the problem area. Moreover, very little cortisone is absorbed into the system as a whole this way, so you don't have to worry about side effects. Medication taken by mouth and absorbed into the bloodstream, however, does travel through your system, and only a very small amount will actually be delivered to the target site. You therefore have to take a larger dose in order to achieve an anti-inflammatory effect at a specific location, and you have to be on the alert for side effects. It just doesn't make sense to take a powerful medication by mouth in order to deliver a tiny portion of it to a specific spot in the body.

If you came to me with, say, a painfully inflamed biceps tendon (bicipital tendinitis), I would inject some cortisone into the area and expect improvement over the next twenty-four to forty-eight hours. This is crucial from a rehabilitation point of view, because once the pain and irritation have settled down, we can start you on a therapeutic exercise program. In the case of bicipital tendinitis, we would want to be sure that your shoulder and arm muscles hadn't tightened up too much, and that you could move your shoulder freely in all directions. If I should choose to inject your tennis elbow, I would follow up with a program of strengthening exercises for the forearm muscles. These muscles would probably have become weaker from not being used as much as usual, so they would have to be built up again. Strengthening them would also cut down on the chances of future episodes of tennis elbow.

The point I want to make is that a cortisone injection is only the beginning of treatment. It must be followed by a program of physical therapy based on a careful analysis of the cause of your injury. Cortisone injections alone will offer temporary relief, but problems are less likely to develop or recur if you combine the injections with a structured exercise program.

I am not in favor, by the way, of giving a *series* of cortisone injections to an inflamed tendon or joint. Too much cortisone can actually weaken the structures you are trying to help. There have been times when I have found it necessary to give a second injection to a particularly troublesome area, but usually the process of inflammation can be controlled sufficiently by a single injection.

CYBEX MACHINE

This relatively new and sophisticated machine can be used both to test and build up muscle strength. At New York Hospital we use it most frequently for the muscles around the knees and shoulders.

As a testing device it can pinpoint deficiencies in the muscle at specific angles or positions along an arc of movement that the physician might not be able to pick up just by applying resistance himself. The machine is hooked up to a computer that will provide a print-out of the results in pounds per square foot for each position of the limb. This information, which is precise and has the patient's "signature" on it, so to speak, can then be used in designing specific rehabilitation programs and monitoring progress.

Often, the use of free weights is sufficient for a strengthening program, but there are certain situations where a Cybex is preferable, such as training a competitive athlete, or building up the knee muscles after a surgical procedure.

The Cybex machine is preset at a certain speed, making it "isokinetic," and is programmed to offer an equal and opposite force to the work being done by your muscles at all points along an arc of motion. Controlling *both* your speed and resistance in this way means that you are unlikely to overdo it and tear your muscles; it also gives the muscles a chance to discharge waste products efficiently, and prevents any undue degree of soreness from developing.

Only Cybex among the various exercise machines provides an equal and opposite force throughout the range and at a controlled speed. With free weights you are making a maximum effort at the beginning of an exercise to overcome inertia. After that, little work is done because momentum carries the weight through the arc of motion. Machines like Nautilus and Universal provide resistance to the work of your muscles throughout the arc of motion, but it is difficult to fine-tune the degree of resistance for each individual. They therefore provide variable resistance and unfortunately the greatest resistance provided by the machine may not coincide with the strongest working capacity of the muscle at a given angle.

Cybex, however, can be set so that a specific muscle or muscle group may be strengthened at the angle or position where it showed up as weakest on the printout.

Cybex machines are still very expensive and not readily available, but they have proven to be useful therapeutic and training devices.

DIABETES

Sugar is the fuel that supplies the energy that makes us work, whether we are writing a letter or splitting wood. But sugar, though it may exist in abundance in the bloodstream, can't do its job unless it is properly regulated and prepared for consumption by the body's cells. A number of hormones, produced by clusters of cells (known as the islets of Langerhans) that are spotted throughout the pancreas, are in charge of this intricate task, and the best known of these hormones is insulin. In simplest terms, insulin turns bloodstream sugar into cell fuel, while a number of other factors in turn control the level of insulin.

When things go wrong with this incredibly delicate metabolic process, there is an excessive residue of sugar; the result is diabetes, a term that covers a number of problems which may have various causes and may create a variety of dangerous side effects on the blood vessels, nerves, kidneys, and heart. Diabetes is a Greek word that means "going through"; the sugar is going through the kidneys, which filter the blood, and on into the urine. Perhaps the best-known form of diabetes is also the least common. This is the type that requires regular insulin injections to keep blood sugar levels in range, and it affects about 500,000 people in this country, many of them children. The cause? A genetic flaw may be involved, for the immune systems of those people who develop this form of the disease seem to respond abnormally to viral attack; in some instances their systems destroy their own insulin-producing cells. This condition of insulin-dependent diabetes is called Type I.

Millions of other Americans—some estimates place the figure at 6 million (while another 5 million are thought to have the disease but not know it)—suffer from a form of diabetes that appears to involve an overtaxing of insulin-producing cells rather than their actual damage. Loss of weight, control of diet, reduction of alcohol consumption, an increase in exercise—any of these measures may be all that is needed (without insulin injections) to help control the problem in most such patients. This condition of *non*insulin-dependent diabetes is called Type II.

Physical activity can presumably have the same beneficial effects on the diabetic patient as it does on anyone else. Knowing how to keep your blood sugar well-controlled *during* periods of exercise is very important because increases in energy expenditure decrease insulin requirements *temporarily.* And you should consult your physician about it. On the other hand there is no evidence that regular exercise affects the function of the intact insulin-producing cells in Type I diabetes directly but it can be helpful in increasing blood flow to the extremities and improving one's general health. Moreover, the long-term effects of regular exercise, especially aerobic exercise, can be very beneficial in mitigating the ill effects of the cardiac or vascular complications that can be so devastating in patients with Type I. As far as we know now, however, regular exercise does not significantly decrease the need for insulin over the long run. This is in contrast to the situation of Type II diabetics who *can* help control their blood sugar levels with regular exercise on a long-term basis.

For years, children with diabetes have been kept from exercising in much the same way that asthmatic children were once overprotected. I think this is a mistake. Once the diagnosis has been made and a child's insulin requirements determined, the parent should sit the child down and explain everything in as much detail as possible, in the course of which it should be made clear that sports are possible, though with certain limitations. It is best, in my opinion, to participate in those sports for which the energy expenditure can be reasonably calculated beforehand. This way the parent can have a good idea of how to adjust the child's insulin dosage to accommodate the body's requirements during periods of increased activity. The physician managing the child's diabetes will help you work out the details. I would not recommend sports that have a high-risk factor for cuts and scratches, such as football and to some extent baseball. Skin abrasions can easily lead to infection, which can be dangerous for insulin-dependent youngsters. The child should also be taught to care immediately for any cuts or blisters that appear on the feet, and to change socks regularly and use antifungal powders.

Basketball, swimming, tennis, and running are all possible for the diabetic child. Not only can the child participate successfully in these activities, but such participation can motivate him or her to a better understanding of the use of insulin and diligence in observing the proper dietary precautions. A physiatrist in cooperation with a pediatric diabetes specialist can work out the proper diabetic and exercise regimen. Usually aerobic exercises are recommended, and recent studies have shown that what is commonly called anaerobic exercise, including weight lifting, can also be beneficial.

ELECTRICAL STIMULATION

The efficiency of electrical stimulation for loosening up tight muscles is well-established. It induces the muscle to contract and relax rhythmically, and it can shorten the time of injury treatment substantially for somebody with very tight muscles. Electrical stimulation involves placing electrodes over the muscles to be treated and delivering a stimulus from a machine called the Medcolator, which plugs into a household outlet and transforms the current into millivolts. There are two main types of stimulation. One, called tetanic, is a constant stimulation that cuts off, then comes on again at regular intervals. The other is the so-called surging type. This form of stimulation gradually increases in strength until the muscle contracts and then abates as the muscle relaxes. Among other forms of electrical stimulation, we sometimes use electrogalvanic stimulation, which is set at a higher frequency and is usually applied to very small areas. Electrical stimulation has no ill effects, and it is painful only if applied over an already irritated nerve. The usual duration of electrical stimulation is about twenty minutes.

If a nerve that supplies a certain muscle is damaged so much that no "active" contraction can be performed—that is, you are unable to contract the muscle at will—then electrical stimulation is definitely indicated. The function of the nerve will take three to four months to return; in the meantime you can maintain the muscle by frequently subjecting it to electrical stimulation. This is important because you don't want the muscle to become fibrotic from disuse. Once there are fibrotic changes in a muscle, it cannot be rehabilitated. It must be pointed out, however, that electrical stimulation does not actually help the nerve recover. The nerve has to recover by itself. When it does, it will find functioning muscle fibers (maintained by electrical stimulation) that can again contract and relax.

If you have a nerve injury, either in your extremities or in your face (most commonly facial palsy), a physiatrist will be able to make a judgment as to whether or not electrical stimulation is needed. If the choice is optional, I strongly advise trying electrical stimulation, because there is no ill effect.

Electrical stimulation to the muscle is also frequently used in sports injuries, especially if an injured extremity has to be placed in a plaster cast. It is then worthwhile having electrodes placed on any muscles immobilized by the cast in order to keep their fibers from deteriorating. But electrical stimulation is not helpful in building strong muscles from already healthy ones. For this you have to perform exercises, preferably against weight resistance.

Electrical stimulation is also used to enhance bone healing in fractures where the two fragments don't unite as expected.

ELECTRODIAGNOSIS

One of the physiatrist's diagnostic tools for ascertaining whether a particular weakness is caused by a muscular problem or by a nerve problem is the electrodiagnostic test, which is divided into a nerve conduction velocity study and a needle electromyography.

The test serves to document and confirm (or rule out) findings that were elicited on physical examination. Measurement of a nerve's conduction velocity—its capacity to conduct an electrical stimulus over a certain distance—can express in numerical terms to what degree a nerve supplying a particular muscle is damaged, something that often cannot be determined by physical examination alone. The way it is done is this: An electrical stimulus is applied to the skin over the course of the nerve in question. An electrode previously placed over the muscle that the nerve is supplying will pick up a signal as soon as the stimulus has reached the muscle. This signal is then shown on a screen displaying a graph that measures the time it took for the stimulus to produce the signal. By measuring the distance between the stimulus and the pick-up electrode, you can calculate the velocity. This test is uncomfortable but not at all painful.

In order to check the electrical "potentials" generated by a muscular contraction, small needle electrodes are inserted into the muscles to be examined. This is called an electromyogram. If there is nerve damage, the muscle potentials will show up as abnormal on the screen. Different types of nerve damage will be reflected in certain patterns. It is also possible to tell whether the injury is recent or old, and it can help to make a prediction as to how long it may take for the nerve to recover, or what the chances of recovery are. In addition, needle electromyography is helpful in distinguishing between weakness caused by nerve damage and weakness caused by muscle disease. Altogether, it helps your physician outline the most appropriate course of treatment.

Many patients are reluctant to undergo an electromyogram because of the needles inserted into the muscles. However frightening this may sound, I can assure you that no injury results, and it is actually not painful if done by an experienced physiatrist or neurologist. If insertion of the needle concerns you, your physician can always use a bit of ethyl chloride spray or some ice to dull the sensation.

Electrodiagnostic studies are no substitute for a careful history and physical examination, however useful they are in the documentation of a working diagnosis. All physiatrists (as well as neurologists) have special training in electrodiagnostic studies.

EXERCISE EQUIPMENT FOR THE HOME

The ingenuity of engineers seems to have no end. While it has been customary for people to go to a gym or health club to use exercise equipment, our modern high-tech era now allows us to have and use similar equipment at home. This can include anything from an exercycle to a treadmill with ergometers or electronic monitoring gadgets. In general, such machines are superbly designed.

There is one general problem, however: Much of this equipment may make you do more than you should at any given time. The condition of our bodies varies from day to day, even during the day, and along with it our capacity for energy expenditure. If you didn't have any monitoring gadgets at home, you would simply stop when you felt tired, and this would, in my opinion, be all to the good. The overall result of a regular exercise program should be a generally improved performance with a *decreased* energy expenditure, a result that is not achieved on a straight-line, upward slope. In reality, there are ups and downs along the way, according to one's daily condition. The human body doesn't perform every day on the same level, even in the case of a highly trained athlete. So home machines, so tempting to use in their immediate and continued availability, should only be used in ways that allow for such human variations, and one should always remember not to push oneself beyond the point of fatigue.

Unfortunately, an increasing number of injuries is being reported from the use of home exercise equipment. None of the injuries are likely to be life-threatening or severe, but long-lasting conditions, such as sciatic nerve root irritation, often called a pinched nerve, are fairly common. As already implied, the fault is not so much with the machine as with the person using it, who is often unaware that he or she is doing anything wrong. Simply not preparing properly for home exercise can be a frequent cause of injury. I think it is therefore worthwhile to consult a physiatrist or knowledgeable physical therapist before you start using such equipment. Together you can evaluate the condition of your muscles and work out some tailored guidelines for your regular use of whatever home equipment you have or desire.

Exercise bicycles are one machine that can provide a good aerobic workout, except for one thing: They may be ridden in such a way (by locking the ankle) that the calf muscle is not used properly and doesn't benefit from increased blood flow and oxygen delivery. Walking and running are good aerobic activities because the heart has to work harder to adequately supply the gastrocnemius (calf) muscle, which uses more oxygen per tissue unit than any other in the body. Bicycling is excellent, too, but to ensure that you use your calves, raise the seat as high as possible so that your leg is fully extended and the ball of your foot just touches the pedal at its lowest point. If you have some form of peripheral vascular disease, this is especially important. And be sure not to move your hips from side to side on the seat as you pedal, or you might develop some back pain. It is always a good idea to have an expert check and make sure that you are using your exercise equipment correctly.

Some machines are designed to help you strengthen certain muscles by your pressing upward against the machine while in a sitting or standing position. This is risky and can cause problems in the lower back or neck. If, for instance, you use the so-called low back machine to strengthen your abdominal muscles with resistance applied against the chest, a lumbar spine condition can easily become aggravated. The same can happen with a rowing machine that drives a large flywheel with air paddles. The faster the wheel goes, the higher the air resistance will be, and the greater the strain on the lower back.

In my opinion, the safest strengthening equipment, especially for people in middle age, is a rope and pulley arrangement with adjustable weights. I use this myself in my backyard. (I use rocks for weights so I don't have to worry about rust!) Like so many busy people, I have no time to go to a gym. I work especially on my upper back and shoulder muscles, mainly to stay in shape for my favorite aerobic activity, swimming.

Home equipment can be helpful and save time, but you should have guidance in using it. Remember to warm up beforehand, to cool down afterward, and not to push yourself beyond the point of fatigue.

FACET SYNDROME

This is a term you may hear from time to time when consulting a physician for low back pain. You should know something about it not because facet syndrome is a common medical problem, but because it is not.

The facet joints are knuckle-sized chunks of bone that lie at the back of the vertebrae and help hold the spine together. They are true joints in that they are covered by the tough tissue that forms the joint capsules and is lubricated by synovial fluid. As you grow older, they, along with most of the other joints in your body, become targets for osteoarthritic changes. It is thought that the changes which affect the facet joints irritate the nerve endings that

supply them, thereby causing pain. These changes can be so severe that they may press on the nerve roots which exit from special openings, or neural foramina, partly bordered by the facet joints. But the real problem with facet syndrome is that the innervation—that is, the nerve supply—is a very complicated one, and it has been shown on anatomical studies to vary greatly from individual to individual. It even varies between the right and left side. It is therefore very difficult to say with any certainty that low back pain is indeed coming specifically from or around the facet joints. I should also emphasize that the pain could be caused by a number of other factors: tight muscles, trigger points, disk disease. An isolated facet joint problem would, in my opinion, be most unlikely.

To my knowledge, there is no reliable specific test to diagnose facet syndrome. I know the diagnosis still pops up on CAT scan and myelogram interpretations from time to time, but as with all kinds of osteoarthritic changes in the spine, facet abnormalities are often not accompanied by any pain.

In the early 1930s, most back problems were attributed to arthritic changes in the facet joints. In 1933, a paper was published reporting a 95-percent cure rate for facet syndrome with Novocain injections. Shortly thereafter, two doctors at Boston's Massachusetts General Hospital were among the first to report that herniated, or "slipped" disks were a common cause of back pain, and from that point on references to facet syndrome all but vanished from the medical literature. For years, disk surgery was the treatment of choice, but, unfortunately, it was found that surgical procedures do not always help, even in the most skilled hands. Then, in the late 1940s, Dr. Hans Kraus, reported that many people with back pain had primarily muscular problems rather than neurological deficits, and thus might benefit from a regular exercise program.

The rate of surgery for slipped disks dwindled after that, and the term "facet syndrome" became popular once more. A high degree of success was attributed to cortisone injections into the facet joints. A review of the literature, however, shows that all treatments for facet syndrome, including surgical removal of the facets, electrical coagulation of the nerves, and cortisone injections, produced an improvement rate of about 33 percent. This is approximately one point above the placebo rate. That is why I am relieved that my neurosurgical colleagues do not attempt any of these procedures.

If you are diagnosed as having the problem, and a surgical intervention of one form or another is suggested, my advice would be to try an exercise program first. Of course, I am prejudiced, but you would not be remiss in consulting a physiatrist who has some expertise in the treatment of low back problems. A facet problem may indeed have triggered a painful reaction in which the muscles went into spasm and caused further pain. Simply by relaxing these muscles and then strengthening them through a very structured exercise program, you have a good chance of decreasing the pain and preventing recurrences. So far, this approach has worked well with patients who have come to me from other physicians with a diagnosis of facet syndrome.

FLATTENED ARCHES

Our arches get flatter as we get older. There is nothing that any of us can do about this. It is impossible to strengthen the arch with any kind of exercise, for there is no specific muscle that holds the arch up; it consists only of ligaments and bones. Therefore, any exercise program, regardless of how well it is designed and how strictly it is adhered to, will not change the actual configuration of the arches. I am not against exercising the feet if it makes you feel better—exercises and massage can help relax your toes and the muscles in your feet and thus improve circulation—but it will not change your anatomical structure.

Some people are born with flat feet and experience little or no pain because of them. If you are such a person and you decide to become a long-distance runner, or participate in any sport that puts a lot of stress on your feet, I would recommend that you invest in custom-fitted arch supports. Go to an expert for such devices—a good orthotist (a specialist in the creation of devices that support the body) or a podiatrist (who knows how to measure and analyze the biomechanics of your foot). Otherwise, you may develop pain in and around your knee, and eventually the hip and low back. This is because the arch is designed to give as your foot hits the ground, and if you have an already flattened arch, impact may be delivered up your leg into your hip and back. Arch supports can help your foot, knee, and leg distribute the punishment created by such repeated pounding.

FROZEN SHOULDER

Keep moving!—that is the essence of the solution to a frozen shoulder problem, a painful and potentially disabling condition that we see frequently at New York Hospital. Not long ago I examined a patient who arrived early one Monday morning without an appointment and insisted on seeing me. When I explained that my schedule was extremely tight, he told me that if I was as good as everyone said, I could take care of him in a minute's time. Well, I couldn't bring myself to turn him away after that bit of flattery, and it's true that it didn't take long to determine that he had a frozen left shoulder as a result of a rotator cuff tear. The tear was something that had happened several months earlier, and the frozen shoulder had developed gradually after that. The irony of this episode, and in a way of all frozen shoulder cases, is that if this blunt and determined patient had used the same resolve for his shoulder problem that he did in dealing with me, he would not have needed my services!

The condition can be caused by almost anything that can trigger pain and discomfort in the shoulder: painting a ceiling, too much gardening or tennis, pulling suitcases from a baggage conveyor belt. Heart attack patients are sometimes afraid to move their shoulders much, so they develop a stiff shoulder from simply lack of movement. Sometimes stress and tension can start things off, and I have even seen cases of a psychosomatic nature: a teacher who ran into the problem when it was time to grade papers; a boss when it was time to trim the staff. Thus, frozen shoulder is really a catchall term and not a specific diagnostic entity. Whatever the underlying cause—a rotator cuff tear, tendinitis, or bursitis, to cite three possibilities—a process known as *adhesive capsulitis* takes place. The sleeve-like capsule that covers the shoulder joint requires movement to stay healthy. When you raise your arm it is much looser, and if you keep your arm at your side long enough, portions of the sleeve can stick together and form little adhesions—hence, adhesive capsulitis.

If you have bursitis, for example, and it hurts to comb your hair or reach up to a shelf, and you use one arm to the exclusion of the other, adhesions in the joint sleeve will begin to form in the less mobile shoulder in about a week. It will then become increasingly difficult for you to move your arm, and if you favor it for another two or three weeks, you will have a serious problem, perhaps even a permanent limitation. It takes a lot of hard work to thaw a frozen shoulder and return it to normal function.

Unfortunately, but not surprisingly, most people don't come to my office with this problem until they have lost substantial movement in their shoulder in all directions. The deltoid muscle, which caps the shoulder, may have undergone serious deterioration. The loss of muscle mass can even be visible when you compare one shoulder to the other. To treat a frozen shoulder, I would try to determine what the underlying cause is: an inflamed bursa or tendon, referred pain from the pancreas or gallbladder, radiating pain from the neck? Then I would try to find out how this all started. And finally, assuming the underlying problem or cause did not require its own separate treatment first, I would outline a special exercise program.

It takes time, two to three months and possibly more, to loosen a shoulder with a carefully planned exercise program. And you have to do your exercises every day. The good news is that if you have a frozen shoulder, you will not develop a second one on the other side: The demands of daily living are sufficient to make you use the other shoulder so much that it can't possibly freeze up!

Immobilization of your shoulder may also develop trigger points in your shoulder muscles, especially in the infraspinatus muscle, which lies directly over the shoulder blade. This may make it difficult to engage in a useful and effective exercise program. I can inject these firm and hardened tangles of muscles, the trigger points, with a mepivacaine hydrochloride and saline solution to break them up, and treat them afterward with electrical stimulation, but trigger point injections alone are not an effective therapeutic program. They can, however, be a very valuable adjunct to the exercise program, and they do speed recovery.

Frozen shoulder is one ailment that calls for the application of heat in order to increase the extensibility of the muscles. You can also use deep heat, like ultrasound, aimed directly into the shoulder joint. In a *chronic* condition, one does not have to worry that heat will increase the swelling, because leakage and accumulation of fluid do not occur when the blood vessels dilate. However, this is not true of *acute* situations. The one consistent and important piece of advice I can give you, is to follow an exercise program on a regular basis and not expect miracles in a week or two, or even a month. Someone may tell you a frozen shoulder can go away by itself, but I have yet to see this happen.

The exercises that follow are helpful in the treatment of frozen shoulder problems. They are the same ones that we prescribe for patients at New York Hospital. Before you consider doing them, however, you should see a physiatrist or orthopedic surgeon and establish a definite diagnosis. Then, if your doctor feels that the exercises are appropriate to your particular disability, you should do them twice a day, morning and night. In doing the exercises, especially when you are stretching your shoulder, you should go to the point of pain and then a little beyond if you can. If pain persists well *after* your session, consult your doctor. The important thing to realize is that you must loosen the adhesions that have formed, and exercises are the best way to do this. You can monitor your progress at home by reaching up as high as you can every day and making a mark on the wall. Remember to breathe normally while you exercise and to relax completely between repetitions. For the best results, it is advisable for a trained therapist to assist you, both in moving your shoulder and in helping you to follow this exercise program or one prescribed by your physiatrist.

EXERCISE 1

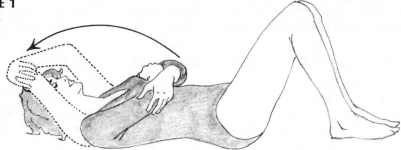

EXERCISE 1

To do this shoulder flexion exercise, sit in a straight-backed chair with your feet flat, or lie on your back on a mat with your knees bent and your feet flat. Firmly cradle your injured arm with the hand of your other arm, then slowly raise both arms over your head as far as possible. Let the uninjured arm do most of the lifting; do not move past the point of pain. Hold your arms in this overhead position for 5 seconds (count to 6), then relax. Repeat this exercise 6 times.

EXERCISE 2

Sit in a straight-backed chair with your feet flat on the floor. Firmly cradle your injured arm with the hand of your other arm. Using the supporting arm, slowly push the injured arm out to that same side. Do not lift your arms upward, just move them sideways in the direction of the injured arm. Hold this position for 5 seconds (count to 6), then relax. Repeat this exercise 6 times.

EXERCISE 2

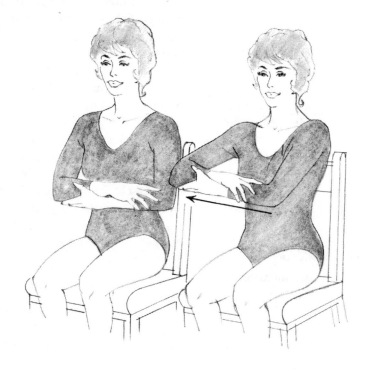

EXERCISE 3

This exercise is designed to stretch the middle trapezius and rhomboid muscles. Sit in a straight-backed chair with your feet flat on the floor. Place the tips of your fingers on your shoulders (right fingers to right shoulder, left fingers to left shoulder). Keeping your hands in place, try to touch your elbows together at shoulder height in front of your chin. Hold this position for 5 seconds (count to 6), then relax. Repeat this exercise 6 times.

EXERCISE 3

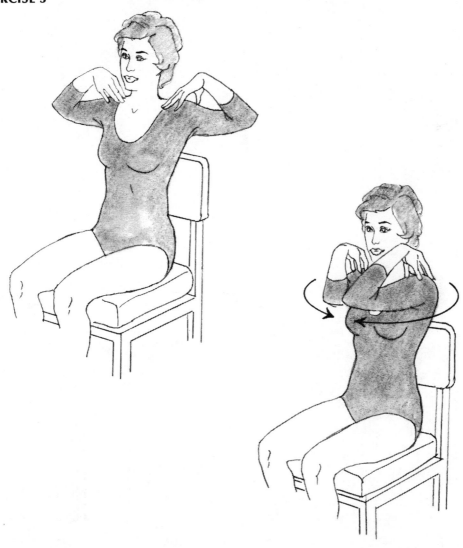

EXERCISE 4

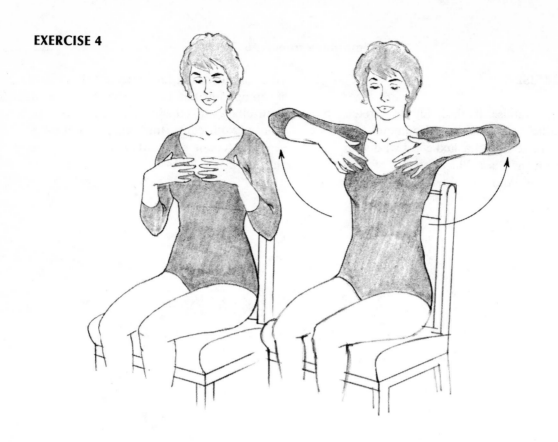

EXERCISE 5

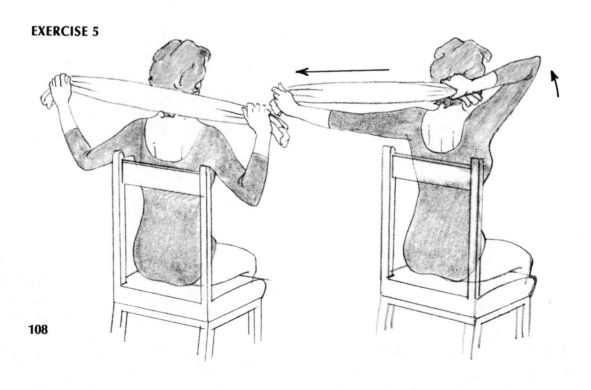

EXERCISE 4

Sit in a straight-backed chair with your feet flat on the floor, or lie on your back on a mat with your knees bent and your feet flat. Place your fingers on your chest as shown in the illustration on page 108, then slowly move your elbows up and out to the sides as far as possible. Be careful not to raise your shoulders. Hold this position for 5 seconds (count to 6), then relax. Repeat this exercise 6 times.

EXERCISE 5

Sit in a straight-backed chair with your feet flat on the floor. Hold a rolled-up towel behind your neck; straighten your uninjured arm and, by doing so, pull the frozen arm up. Attempt to point the elbow of the frozen arm toward the ceiling until you feel pain. Hold this position for 5 seconds (count to 6), then relax. Repeat this exercise 6 times.

EXERCISE 6

This exercise will stretch the shoulder. Sit in a straight-backed chair, or on a stool, with your feet flat on the floor. Raise your arms over and behind your head, firmly grip the elbow of your injured arm with your other hand. Gently pull your elbow toward your uninjured side as far as possible. Remain in this position for 5 seconds (count to 6), then relax. Repeat this exercise 6 times.

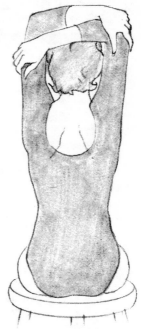

EXERCISE 6

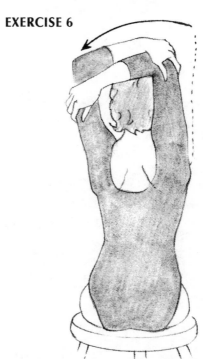

EXERCISE 7

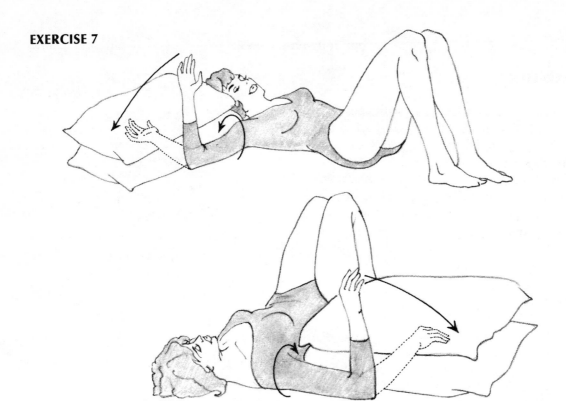

EXERCISE 8

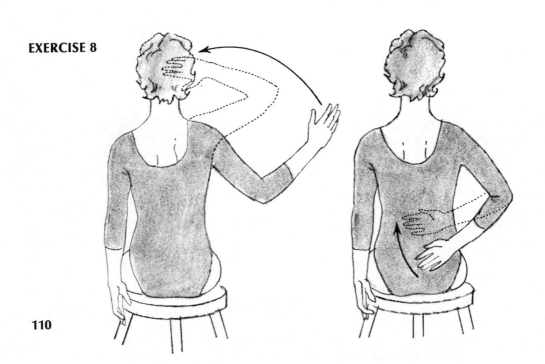

EXERCISE 7

To do this shoulder rotation exercise you will need two pillows (if you feel no pain while exercising with two pillows, then use only one). Lie on your back on a mat with your knees bent and feet slightly apart and flat on the floor. The pillows should be on the injured side, next to your head. Slide your injured arm out to the side, until it is in line with your shoulder. Bend your elbow to 90 degrees, raising your forearm upright; rotate your arm at the shoulder so that the top of your forearm rests on the pillows without pain. Keep your shoulder flat on the floor. Hold this position for 5 seconds (count to 6), then relax. Repeat this exercise 6 times.

Next, move the pillows next to your ribs on the injured side, and place your injured arm in the starting position as above—with the elbow bent at a 90-degree angle. Rotate your arm at the shoulder so that the underside of your forearm rests on the pillows without pain. Keep your shoulder flat on the floor. Hold this position for 5 seconds (count to 6), then relax. Repeat this exercise 6 times.

EXERCISE 8

This exercise is for shoulder rotation. Sit up straight on a stool with your feet flat on the floor and your uninjured arm hanging down at your side. Lift your injured arm, keeping the elbow out to the side, and try to touch the back of your head with the palm of your hand. If no pain occurs, try to touch the lower part of your neck. Hold this position for 5 seconds (count to 6), then relax. Repeat this exercise 6 times.

Next, try to touch your lower spine with the back of your hand. Slide your hand up along the spine as far as possible. Hold this position for 5 seconds (count to 6), then relax. Repeat this exercise 6 times.

EXERCISE 9

To do this shoulder rotation exercise, sit up straight on a stool with your feet flat on the floor. Place both hands behind your back and grasp the wrist of your injured arm with your other hand. Letting the uninjured arm do most of the work, slowly slide both hands up your spine toward the shoulder blades as far as possible without straining or pain. Hold this position for 5 seconds (count to 6), then relax. Repeat this exercise 6 times.

EXERCISE 9

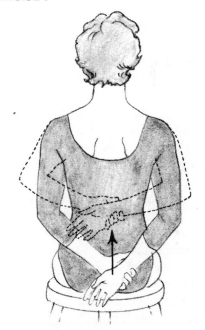

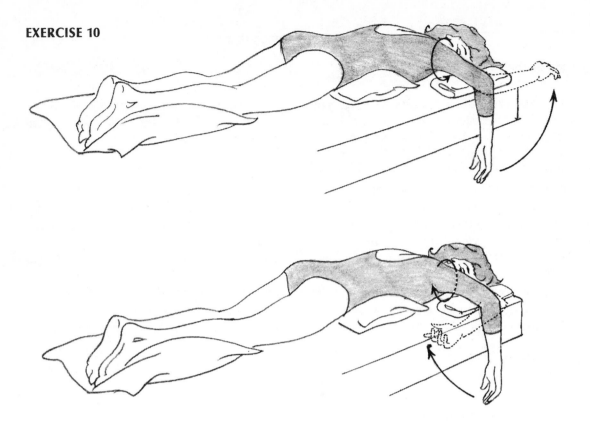

EXERCISE 10

This shoulder rotation exercise should be done lying prone on a bed, with pillows under your abdomen and ankles. Slide your injured arm up to shoulder height and let it hang over the edge of the bed at the elbow. Place a rolled-up towel under the upper arm. Then, by rotating at the shoulder, roll your arm forward so that your hand raises toward your head. Hold this position for 5 seconds (count to 6), then relax. Repeat this exercise 6 times. Next, rotate your shoulder again, but this time roll your arm backward, so that your hand points toward your feet. Hold this position for 5 seconds (count to 6), then relax. Repeat this exercise 6 times.

GOLFER'S ELBOW

Like tennis elbow, this term refers to tendon irritation, either at a muscle-tendon junction in the upper forearm or where the tendon is anchored to the bone. Unlike tennis elbow, which usually causes pain on the outer side of the elbow, golfer's elbow most often affects the inner aspect, at about the elbow crease where a tendon binds the forearm muscles to the bony promontory known as the medial epicondyle. Contraction of the wrist-flexing muscles at the end of the golf swing causes the fraying or irritation of the tendon that produces the pain.

A condition like golfer's elbow can be caused by other activities besides golf.

Gripping the handles of a bicycle can do it, or digging in the garden, or using a terminal wrist slap at the end of your tennis serve. In the 1900s, what is now known as golfer's elbow was more commonly found among those tennis players who often hit their forehand ground strokes with the racquet head down.

It is also possible for golfers to develop tennis elbow pain, a condition caused by quick extension of the left wrist (in a right-handed person) at the end of or during follow-through.

Whatever the cause, if you have golfer's elbow, I suggest you do the exercises described in the Tennis Elbow section. Be sure to emphasize the second exercise, which is especially helpful for golfer's elbow.

GROIN PULL

This is a common but misleading term. The muscles involved in a so-called groin pull are actually the hip adductor muscles, which are located on the inside of the thigh and enable you to bring your legs together. The damage does not directly involve the groin area itself, which is technically the junction between the abdomen and thigh. Some injuries to the adductors are relatively minor, but others can be long lasting and difficult to treat.

In most cases of groin pull, a few fibers in the hip adductor muscles are overstretched and a few others ripped. If clinical examination indicates this type of problem, then it shouldn't take more than a few weeks to rehabilitate the injury. You

simply avoid overexertion of the muscle and try some gentle limbering and stretching exercises a week or two after the injury, while healing is taking place. If the injury occurs higher up, however, where the tendon is attached to the pelvic bone, then the damage can be very painful and similar to what happens in acute tennis elbow, where the area beneath the tendon becomes irritated and inflamed. Such a situation will require more care and time. You may have to use a cylindrical brace around the thigh for four to six weeks if you want to participate again in such sports as racquetball or tennis.

In general, if you participate in activities that require special exertion of the hips—tennis, jogging, soccer, skiing—it is crucial that you loosen your adductor muscles before every session. If you don't, you increase your chances of incurring this painful injury. Kicking a soccer ball with the inside of your foot is a common way to rip an adductor muscle. Golfers can also tear the hip adductors by overstretching at the top of the backswing, especially when their feet are solidly spiked into the ground. You can even tear your adductors with an angry sideways kick at a suitcase or a door that won't open.

In severe cases I recommend walking on crutches for a week or two so the injured muscle remains free to heal. The next step is a carefully structured program of physical therapy, first to loosen and then to strengthen the muscles involved. The real dangers here are that the abductor muscles, which oppose the adductors, will become weak from lack of use; that the hip will lose its range of motion; and that the injured adductor muscle will tighten as it heals. If you don't do anything to rehabilitate the adductor muscle, it will heal on its own, but you'll still have a strong chance of suffering another pull; the muscle will be tight from healing and ripe for tearing.

The exercises that follow will help to limber, stretch, and strengthen your hip adductor muscles whether they are healthy or recovering from injury. Stretching is crucial, because damaged fibers become shorter as they heal. It is extremely important, however, to wait at least two or three weeks to do more than the limbering exercises. Your physiatrist or orthopedic surgeon can advise you on this. When doing stretching exercises, stretch until you feel the beginnings of a pull. Hold at that point and breathe slowly while the tension eases, then try to go a *little* bit further. Be careful not to overstretch; this can rerupture fibers, especially in the early stages of healing. You may want to apply ice three times a day for the first thirty-six to seventy-two hours, and then apply heat to improve circulation and remove waste products. Re-

member to breathe normally while exercising and to relax completely between repetitions.

EXERCISE 1

Lie on your uninjured side, knees slightly bent. Slide the heel of the injured side along the shin of the uninjured one, up to the knee. Lift the knee on the injured side, rotating the hip joint, and hold for 5 seconds (count to 6); return to the original position. Repeat 5 to 6 times.

EXERCISE 2

Lie on your back with knees bent and feet flat on the floor. Starting with your uninjured leg, hook that foot behind your other heel. Let the uninjured leg fall gently to the outside without straining. Hold it there for 15 seconds (count to 18). Return to the starting position, relax, and repeat with the injured leg. Repeat 3 times in the beginning, and increase by one repetition each day to a total of 5.

EXERCISE 1

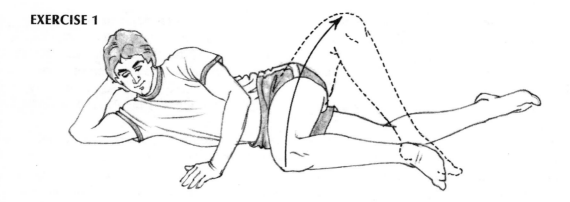

EXERCISE 2

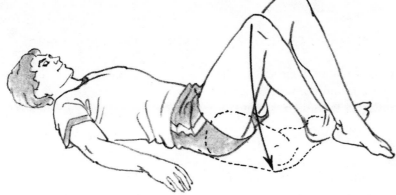

EXERCISE 3

Sit on the floor with your legs outstretched to form a V. Bend your knees and move your feet in toward your body until the soles of your feet are together. Grasp your ankles, rest your elbows on the inside of your knees and bend over slightly so that your elbows gently push your knees toward the floor. Hold this for as long as is comfortable, up to 15 seconds (count to 18). Do not force the movement or bounce. Release and relax. Repeat 3 times to begin with, and increase by one repetition each day up to a total of 5 repetitions.

EXERCISE 3

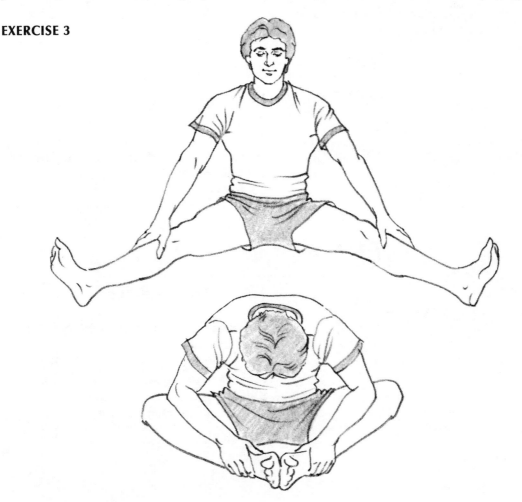

Once these three stretching exercises can be done without pain and the injured area is no longer tender to the touch, strengthening exercises may be started. You should consult your physiatrist or orthopedic surgeon to determine when to start the next two exercises. Do them twice a day, morning and night.

EXERCISE 4

Sit in a straight-backed chair with your feet flat on the floor; place a soft beach ball between your knees. Compress the ball with your knees and hold each compression for 5 seconds (count to 6), then relax for 3 seconds (count to 4). Start with 3 repetitions and gradually build up to 12.

EXERCISE 4

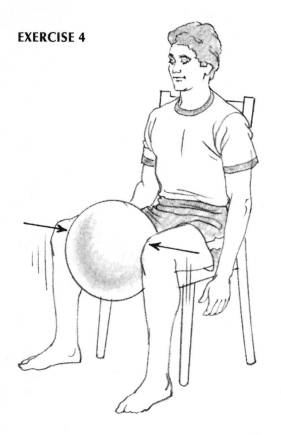

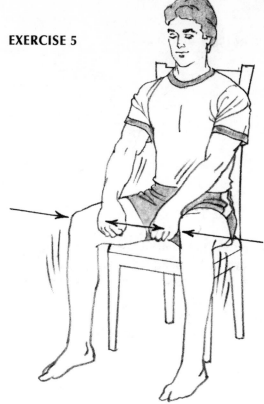

EXERCISE 5

EXERCISE 5

Sit in a straight-backed chair with your feet flat on the floor and shoulder-width apart. Make your hands into fists and place them on the inside of each knee. As you push out with your fists, try to bring your knees together. Hold at a point of tension for 5 seconds, then relax. Start off with 8 repetitions and increase over a week's time to 15.

HAMSTRING PULL

Two natural but quite different forces control body movement. One is gravity, the other is the capacity of muscle fibers to contract at the command of a motor nerve. Raise your right arm to shoulder height and let it drop. Down it goes, smack against your thigh, thanks to the pull of gravity. Lift that same arm back up again, against the pull of gravity, and dozens of muscles in your arm, shoulder, back, and chest contract to do the job.

This is not only a remarkably intricate sequence, it works. Yet to deliver movements large or small—to move a limb up and down or clockwise and counterclockwise—the body harnesses opposing pairs of muscles; one contracts while the other relaxes, and vice versa. Certain diseases—Parkinson's for one—disrupt this measured interaction of muscle against muscle and produce a slow, hesitant motion. If you move the arm of a Parkinson's patient, you will feel a cogwheel-like resistance instead of a smooth, integrated motion. Muscle pairs can create problems, too. For example, one muscle may be stronger than its opposing partner and overpower it, or, because of strain or a fall, a muscle may contract so swiftly that its partner can't relax in time. When this happens, the muscle that was supposed to relax can tear.

This is exactly what occurs when you pull a hamstring. The hamstring muscles fill the back of the thigh above the knee and work in tandem with the quadriceps muscle in the front of the thigh. Together they form the body's most powerful partnership. The quads lift and straighten out or extend the knee, the hamstrings bend the knee. Sprinters, straining to break records, and baseball players, dashing to first base, often tear hamstrings. But so can anyone. It's not hard at all, especially if you play tennis without warming up, hike over rough ground, or trip and fall on a bumpy lawn.

However the injury may come to pass,

you will know it. It will feel as if a stray bullet has hit you, or somebody has clipped you in the back of the thigh with a tennis racquet. Should you remain uncertain whether you've pulled a hamstring, there is a simple test you can perform on yourself or with the help of a friend. Lie on your stomach, bend the knee of your injured leg halfway, and look or feel for two hard tendons thrusting up just above the back of your knee. These connect the hamstring muscles to the knee, and if one of them is sagging or not visible in comparison with your other leg, you can be sure that you have ripped a hamstring. Still, it is always worthwhile to get confirmation from a physiatrist or orthopedic surgeon.

I know exactly what a torn hamstring feels like—I ripped one quite badly last summer while playing tennis. It happened in an instant when I lost my balance and pitched forward. The next thing I felt was a pop in the back of my thigh. Then the area went numb, and I knew what had happened.

Let me tell you what I did to treat the tear. Though it's not exactly a standard approach, it should help you understand the injury and the rationale behind the more conventional therapies.

After cooling off, I went swimming in Long Island Sound, which was freezing. The chilly waters helped dampen the pain and reduce the swelling caused by the rupture that had occurred at the muscle-tendon connection. During the months that followed, despite well-meaning suggestions from colleagues that I undergo surgery, I used electrical stimulation to relax the damaged muscles. And I sat on cold pack after cold pack for twenty minutes at a time, usually while I talked with patients. Every day I stretched my hamstrings carefully. But the tear was a bad one (when I tried the test mentioned earlier, I could feel no anatomical structure at all popping up at the back of my knee), and it continued to bother me all summer. I limped, I stretched, I applied cold, and I waited for improvement.

Finally, in the fall, I had to fly to Switzerland on business. This was just about the time for me to begin strengthening my injured hamstring muscles—the tendons were becoming visible again and I was having less pain. With a wonderful view of the majestic Swiss mountains from my hotel room, I couldn't bear the thought of doing strengthening exercises alone in my room, so I decided to do my rehabilitation by walking up a mountain, which would strengthen my quadriceps primarily, and to a lesser degree my hamstrings. At a certain point I could then start going downhill, too, which would make my hamstrings work even harder.

At first I hiked short distances uphill and had to hitch rides back down because my hamstrings were too tight and painful to manage downhill walking. Every day I climbed higher and higher until finally I could take the cable car back down from the top. My quads did the hard work, driving my legs up the incline, but my healing hamstrings had to work, too. Finally I was ready to tackle the downhill slope, and gradually the hamstring muscles, already healed and stretched, were sufficiently in balance with my quadriceps. By the time I returned to New York, my leg was completely restored.

When faced with a hamstring pull, the important things to know are: one, the injured fibers will heal naturally on their own if given the chance; and two, this is an injury that will take time to rehabilitate, especially if the tear is substantial—not a couple of weeks, but six weeks to two or three months.

One of the major problems with hamstring pulls, as with other muscle tears, is that the torn fibers, in the process of healing, become shorter. Thus, what may feel like a healed leg may indeed be healed, but it will still be vulnerable to retearing when you stretch or contract it suddenly. Torn muscle fibers must first heal, and then they have to be stretched and strengthened so that they regain their pretear level of fitness.

If I have a patient who is young and on the reckless side, I will order him onto crutches for two to three weeks after injury. This will give the fibers a chance to begin healing. You may want to consider doing the same thing if you are an unusually active person. And then when you and your doctor are reasonably sure that healing has occurred—say, four to six weeks—you should begin stretching and strengthening not just the injured muscle but your quadriceps as well. Remember, if you have been protecting your hamstrings, your quads have been inactive, too, and the quadriceps are highly susceptible to wasting away and getting weak.

In building up both your hamstrings and quads, you basically have to do what I did in Switzerland: stretch and strengthen both muscle groups at the same time. Four exercises are explained below. The first two are often used by runners and joggers to stretch their hamstrings before workouts.

They are appropriate for you as a way to ease your hamstrings back into working condition. But be careful. If you exert too much force stretching, you run the risk of tearing the same fibers again, especially in the early stages of healing. Stretch until you feel the beginnings of a pull but no strain or pain. Hold at that point and breathe slowly while the tension eases, and then try to go a *little* further. Remember to breathe regularly while exercising and to relax completely between repetitions. The second two exercises are designed to help strengthen your hamstrings.

It is important that your doctor decide when you are ready to begin stretching and toning up your injured hamstrings. It would also be worthwhile to see a physiatrist who can guide you and your physical therapist through your period of rehabilitation, and determine how frequently you should do the exercises.

EXERCISE 1

Lie on your back with your arms relaxed at your sides, your knees bent, and your feet slightly apart and flat on the floor. Slowly push the small of your back into the floor while bringing the knee of your injured leg toward your chest, foot flexed. Straighten the injured leg up slowly until the knee is extended (you may have to lower your leg to achieve this). You should feel a pull in the back of your thigh. Hold for 15 seconds (count to 18), then slowly lower your leg and relax for 10 seconds (count to 12). Do 6 repetitions.

EXERCISE 1

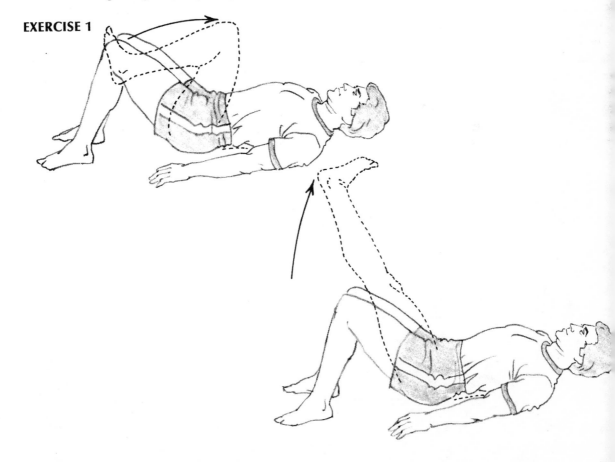

EXERCISE 2

Do not do this exercise if you have a problem with your back. Sit on the floor, leaning against a wall, and stretch your legs straight out. Cross your left ankle over your right (keep both relaxed and your legs fully extended throughout the exercise). Bend forward slowly from the waist, reaching toward your ankles. Do not bounce or jerk. You should feel the pull on the underside of your bottom thigh. Hold this position for 15 seconds (count to 18). Relax for 5 seconds (count to 6). Make sure that all tension has left your muscles before each repetition. After 6 repetitions, reverse and cross your right leg over your left, and proceed as before.

EXERCISE 2

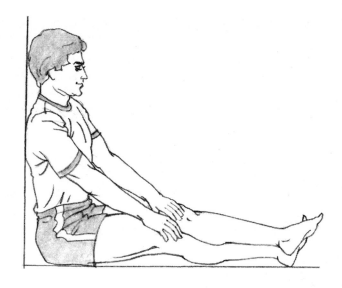

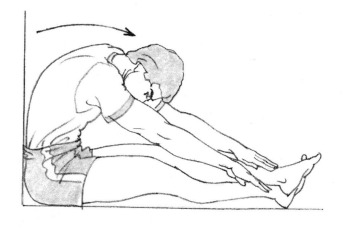

EXERCISE 3

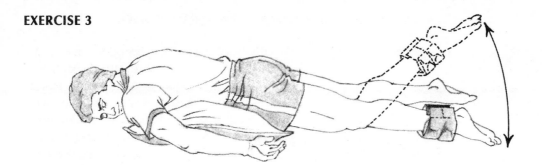

EXERCISE 3

This exercise will help strengthen your hamstrings. Lie on your stomach with a pillow under your abdomen and a 2-pound weight on your ankle. Slowly bend your knee and raise your lower leg to a 45-degree angle; hold this position for 5 seconds (count to 6), then come down. Another way of doing this exercise is to use the full 5 seconds (count to 6) to flex the knee, before coming back down again. Relax all tension in your muscles between each repetition. If 2-pound weights are too much, start with 1-pound weights. Gradually work up to 12 repetitions, then add another pound, drop to 8 repetitions, and work back up to 12. Try to work up to 20-pound weights. Exercise both legs once a day.

EXERCISE 4

This exercise is designed to stretch the quadriceps and strengthen the hamstring muscle at the same time. Lie on your stomach with a pillow under your abdomen and a 1- or 2-pound weight on your ankle. Slowly bend the knee and raise your lower leg to a 90-degree angle, then slowly raise the thigh and hold for 5 seconds (count to 6); or you can use the full 5 seconds (count to 6) to lift and lower your hip. Gradually work up to 12 repetitions, then add another pound, drop down to 8 repetitions, and work back up to 12. Do this exercise once a day.

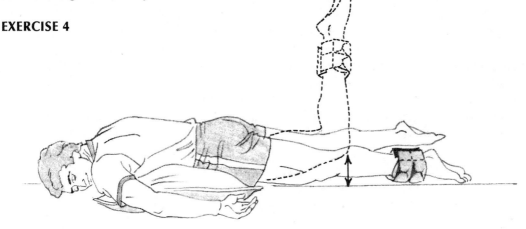

HEEL SPURS AND PLANTAR FASCIITIS

This is a condition resulting from continued wear and tear on the bottom of the heel and on the ligament known as the plantar fascia, which is anchored there. This strong fiber stretches forward from the heel, then branches and hooks to each of the toes. The ligament helps firm up the bottom of the foot and tightens the structure of the arch. Excessive pounding on concrete or asphalt, feet that tend to turn inward, and shoes or sneakers with stiff soles all contribute to the development of a "plantar fasciitis," which is often a forerunner of heel spur formation.

How does this painful condition come about? Most commonly the ligament rubs over and irritates the bone of the heel. The heel bone's response to this irritation is inflammation, increased calcification, and ultimately the formation of a hook or spur at the site. This spur, which shows up clearly on X-rays, in turn adds to the fraying of the ligament that triggered its formation in the first place.

Diagnosis of heel spurs is easy because few other problems cause such intense pain and tenderness in the heel area. Manual pressure on the ball of the heel and X-ray examinations are usually sufficient to make the identification; unlike the case of low back pain, X-ray findings are directly related to the patient's pain. Ice, aspirin, or other anti-inflammatory medications and, if you are a runner, time off from pounding the pavements are advisable initially. If the pain is very severe, you may have to use crutches for a few days. Otherwise a heel cup that fits into the shoe may provide adequate relief; the cup redistributes the forces around the heel and, as such, puts less pressure on the site of the spur. You should also consider footgear with slightly raised heels that will shift your weight forward and thus reduce the impact on the heels of your feet as you run or walk.

In cases of acute inflammation, steroids may need to be injected right into the area where the spur comes off the heel bone. This should then be followed by phonophoresis—the application of cortisone cream in conjunction with ultrasound-wave treatment. The treatment is supposed to drive the cortisone cream into the area of inflammation around the spur, and the ultrasound-waves create deep heat in the surrounding tissue.

Surgical removal of bony spurs used to be recommended, but I've never seen any definite, long-lasting beneficial effect from such a procedure. The bony spur is all too likely to grow back again. Sometimes splitting the plantar fascia can be helpful—the spur is then able to slip through without causing any irritation. In any case, if you leave the spur where it is it does no harm. You are usually better off leaving it alone and simply taking care of the inflammation and making some careful adjustments in your shoes. With time, an improvement is usually realized and you can resume your normal athletic activities.

HIGH-HEEL SHOES

The questions I am asked most frequently about women's footwear are: (1) Will wearing high heels hurt my back or spine? (2) Can high heels damage my feet and toes? (3) If I have flat feet, can I wear high heels? (4) How long should I wear high heels at a time? The answers to these questions are relatively simple: (1) yes and no; (2) yes; (3) yes; and (4) as long as you have to, but change whenever you can.

The facts behind these answers, at least based on my experience, are a bit complicated. For many women, wearing heels even for relatively long periods of time won't cause low back or spinal problems. For others, however, the postural changes caused by two- or three-inch heels can bring pain and misery. Those most likely to suffer are women with weak abdominal and tight hip flexor muscles. That's because these muscles help to align the back and pelvis, and when they get flabby the pelvis will tilt forward, exaggerating the curve in the lower spine (hyperlordosis) and setting the stage for painful muscle spasms in the lower back. Wearing high heels itself tilts the pelvis forward and contributes to this unfavorable situation.

The pelvis-back relationship is hard to measure because the alignment of the spine changes subtly when the muscles around it respond to touch. However, researchers have managed to outwit the "shifty" back. Instead of measuring it, they photographed profile silhouettes of heel wearers and found that high heels did indeed increase the lordosis of the spines of those with the weakest abdominal muscles. So the message is clear: If you wear heels (whether you have back problems or not), work to keep your abdominals tight and hip flexors stretched.

High heels do put more stress on your feet and toes: they function rather like a wedge or ramp, tipping your weight forward and down on to the fragile trapezoid formed by the ball of your foot, your toes, and the sides of your shoes. This pressure sometimes traumatizes the metatarsal bones, which lead from the arch of your foot to the toe joints. Repeated impact may cause osteoarthritic changes in these bones or podiatric problems in the toes themselves. On the outside of the big toe the result may be a condition known as a hallus valgus—the scientific name for common bunions. Furthermore—and heel wearers often forget this—high heels add enormously to your chances of twisting or spraining an ankle, especially when you walk on rough surfaces and in bad weather.

Flat feet, or feet in which the arch has gradually settled with the passage of time, are no more vulnerable to the stresses and strains of high heels than are normal feet. In fact, most people with flat feet, unless they are long-distance runners, don't usually experience serious problems.

Wearing high heels is a personal and oftentimes business-related decision. Thus, the best advice I can give anyone who chooses to wear heels, for whatever the reason, is: Don't wear heels any more than you have to, and if you can, change the type of shoe you wear and vary the heights of your heels as often as possible.

One of the great attractions of high heels, of course, is that they appear to add slimness and elegance to your legs. But there are other ways of shaping a leg, and walking is one of them. Walking up hills is effective, and so is climbing stairs. Stair climbing not only stretches the heel cord (the length of tendon and muscle that runs along the back of your leg and is shortened by wearing heels), it also strengthens the quadriceps, thereby shaping the thighs and strengthening the buttock muscles.

To get the most out of stair climbing, put your hands behind your back and touch each step with the ball of your foot, allowing the heel to sink slightly. Then lift your body on up to the next step and onto the ball of your other foot. Do this slowly and carefully, and no more than two or three flights at a time. When you put your hands behind your back, you are eliminating the balancing action of the arms while you walk up the stairs, transferring it instead to your calf and thigh muscles as an additional strengthening component.

There are a number of things you can do to ease your aching toes, arches, feet, and legs after a long day on heels. Simply removing your shoes and walking around in bare feet can be a help in starting the process of stretching the heel cord.

There are three exercises that will help ease the tightness in your heel cords. The first is walking upstairs as described above. The other two are stretches.

EXERCISE 1

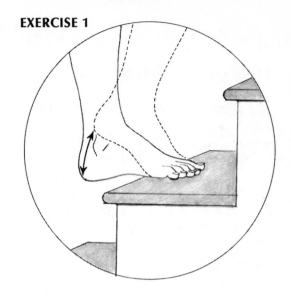

EXERCISE 1

As you walk up stairs, touch the tread with the ball of your foot and let your heel go down before you step up to the next stair. Use each stair to lift the weight of your body up to the next. This stretches and strengthens the calf muscles.

The remaining two exercises are stretches only. In both, stretch until you feel the beginnings of a pull. Hold at that point and slowly breathe in and out a few times while the tension eases, then try to go a little bit further. Remember to breathe regularly while stretching, and to completely relax between repetitions. Hold the stretch for 15 seconds, then relax for 3 to 4 seconds.

EXERCISE 2

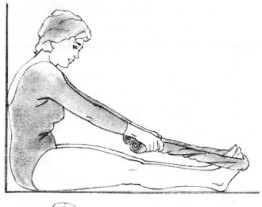

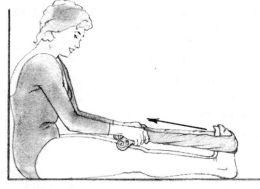

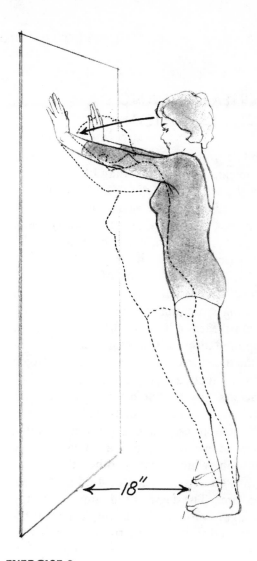

EXERCISE 2

Sit on the floor and extend your legs in front of you, ankles together. Reach forward and hook a rolled towel around the balls of your feet. Keeping your knees straight, pull back firmly on the towel until you feel tension in the back of your lower legs. Hold for 15 seconds (count to 18), then release. Relax for 3 to 4 seconds (count to 4 or 5). Do 5 or 6 repetitions.

EXERCISE 3

This is a traditional runner's exercise, and you have probably seen people doing it. Stand about 18 to 24 inches from a wall,

EXERCISE 3

feet together and flat on the floor; press your palms against the wall. Bend your elbows and lean your upper body into the wall. Be sure to keep your heels flat on the floor and your knees straight. Do not arch your back. You will feel the pull at the back of your legs. Hold for 15 seconds (count to 18), then release. Relax for 3 to 4 seconds (count to 4 or 5). Do 5 or 6 repetitions.

125

IRRITATION AND INFLAMMATION

Should you suffer from a musculoskeletal problem, you will more than likely encounter the terms "irritation" and "inflammation." Both are used for diagnostic purposes, though they are usually quite nonspecific. Just about any part of the body can become irritated or inflamed.

Irritation can be part of a mechanical process, such as the friction caused by two moving structures within a joint rubbing against each other, or the pressure of a ruptured disk pressing against a nerve root. Sometimes irritation has an immunologic source, such as in rheumatoid arthritis. Bacterial toxins that have entered a joint cavity can also act as irritants.

Irritation can then set off a complex chain of events known as an inflammatory reaction, which, among other things, involves an accumulation of fluid in a localized area. The degree of inflammation may be highly variable. For example, if your biceps tendon becomes irritated from overuse after several sets of tennis, the tendon and tendon sheath will swell with an increased fluid content and become very painful. This is generally a low-grade inflammation. A joint cavity can also become inflamed from overuse, even if the joint structure is sound to start with. A joint affected by osteoarthritis is even more susceptible to "flare-ups" because the glistening cartilage, made rough and uneven by osteoarthritis, becomes a source of friction when other structures come in contact with it. In rheumatoid arthritis, joints can be damaged by an overgrowth of synovial tissue, which also sets up an irritative mechanism for inflammation. The joint becomes inflamed and swollen because the production of synovial fluid goes into high gear as a form of protection against the friction between moving parts, or against some other source of irritation. The area becomes swollen, and this is often visible as a bulge under the skin. It may also become warm and red from the increased metabolic activity in the area, and it can be very painful from the pressure on involved and surrounding structures.

When a joint becomes acutely inflamed, the application of heat will only increase the fluid volume and thus cause more pain. Ice does the opposite, and that is why ice applications are recommended in such instances. (See Cold and Heat Treatments.)

ISOMETRIC, ISOTONIC, AND ISOKINETIC EXERCISE

The term "isometric exercise" applies to a muscle contraction that does not visibly move a joint through an arc of motion—for instance, if one just tightens up the muscles. The muscle fibers contract, and therefore the muscle belly increases in diameter. The application of isometric exercise is limited. Its main advantage is in rehabilitation, where it is necessary to avoid any possible damage to the joints, and it can even be practiced with inflamed joints. It does somewhat increase muscular strength, though usually not observably, and it helps to retard muscular atrophy. It can also be beneficial in decreasing any swelling, since the process of contraction and relaxation removes fluid. The disadvantage of isometric exercise is that it can increase blood pressure. It is also extremely boring!

Another fairly recent development is isotonic exercise, frequently referred to as progressive resistive exercise, or training against resistance. Isotonic exercises maintain the same constant tension on the muscle throughout the whole range of movement. They are generally divided into concentric muscle loading and eccentric muscle loading. If, in a sitting position, I put weights around the ankles and straighten the knee, I am concentrically loading the quadriceps. If, next, I slowly bend the knee, that is eccentric loading. In concentric loading, there is an actual shortening of the muscle accompanied by movement of the joint. Both concentric and eccentric loading are features of Nautilus and Universal machines, but they can also be achieved, perhaps less precisely, with free weights. Eccentric loading is used to lengthen the muscle by gradually controlling weight resistance with the muscle contracted as it relaxes. But don't cheat: You must perform the complete arc of motion each time to render the exercises effective.

The third and most recently developed resistive exercise is called isokinetic (see also Cybex Machine). The principle is to maintain a fixed speed with a variable resistance throughout the individual's range of motion. The velocity remains at a preselected range, and the resistance varies to exactly match the force being applied all along the range of motion. Isokinetic exercise allows for maximal dynamic loading—that is, for maximal resistance in exercising throughout the full range of motion at a fixed velocity. Isokinetic and isotonic exercises offer different routes to the same goals: strengthening of the muscles.

JOINT CLICKING AND CRACKING

When people hear their joints clicking or cracking under continual movement, they often jump to the conclusion that they are afflicted with a severe form of arthritis. This is not necessarily the case. A clicking hip, for instance, can be caused by the so-called ilio-tibial band moving over a bone. This band is not, per se, a separate anatomical structure. It belongs to a muscle on the outside of your thigh called the tensor fascia lata, and its uppermost attachment site is on the pelvic bone. It then passes over the hip joint and attaches again just below the knee. If the hip flexor muscle is very tight, the band will click as it moves over the bone, similar to a very tight rope moving over a rounded object; it doesn't glide over, but kind of snaps along. When you bend the thigh and then straighten it out again, the tendon snaps over the pelvic bone underneath. This sometimes occurs in a person who has suffered a pelvic fracture that has not healed altogether symmetrically. There is nothing dangerous about it, and with the proper stretching exercises the clicking will disappear.

People also often complain about cracking sounds in their neck. Again, in many instances this is simply caused by very tight neck muscles, and loosening up of the neck muscles usually eliminates the clicking or cracking. In the knee joints, clicking may come from some unevenness on the inner side of the kneecap; as the kneecap glides over the lower end of the thigh bone, it makes a crackling sound. But again, if the quadriceps and hip flexor muscles are well-stretched, the clicking can be lessened or go away completely.

Of course, the actual cracking of the joints *can* be caused by osteoarthritis, but even this cracking is usually aggravated by tight muscles and their corresponding tendon. Since you cannot stretch a tendon but can stretch a muscle, it is always a good idea to work at keeping the muscles loose, and thereby reducing the tension on the tendon.

The condition known as trigger finger—a locked finger that can only be opened by force—also belongs in the category of clicking joints. In this case, though, the tendon gets stuck in the surrounding tendon sheath because of unevenness inside the sheath, usually in the form of small inflammatory nodules. The irritation of a trigger finger can be alleviated with the application of ultrasound and therapeutic exercises. Sometimes, however, a trigger finger has to be operated on. This should be done only if the function of the hand is impaired.

You may find the clicking of a joint (loose cartilage particles can make a similar sound) noticeable only at the beginning of a motion. If you then move the joint a few times to loosen up the muscles, the clicking disappears. If it doesn't, consult a physiatrist or rheumatologist and they will advise you about what exercises to do. The exercises should be shown to you and done together with a physical therapist, and you should be reevaluated two or three times over the next few weeks to make sure you are doing them correctly.

KNEE JOINT AND LIGAMENT INJURIES

Despite the power of our muscles and the strength of our bones, the human body would be immobile without joints. These intricate and often vulnerable intersections of two or more bones make the spectrum of human movement possible, from the visual magic of a ballerina's pirouette to the power of a baseball player's swing.

Not all joints are alike. Perhaps the easiest to understand is the hinge joint, which permits motion in two directions on a single plane. This means that the joint may open (extend) or close (flex) but not move much from side to side or rotate. The elbow and finger joints are examples of this type of connection. Ball-and-socket joints, found in the hip and shoulder, permit not only rotation but movement in a variety of directions or planes.

The knee is really a combination joint with a primarily hingelike action but also the ability to rotate inward slightly. Its construction is intricate, and the pounding it sometimes takes makes it highly susceptible to injury. It uses muscle, ligament, tendon, and cartilage to anchor and cushion its remarkably versatile capabilities.

Two major leg bones meet at the knee: the shinbone, or tibia, and the thighbone, or femur. The connection they form is rather like two very shallow ball-and-socket joints set side by side. The top of the shinbone contains two slight hollows, and the end of the thighbone a pair of rounded bony protrusions. These fit together, and the circular rim that surrounds them is padded with cartilage, known as the meniscus, which helps distribute weight and keeps the joints from rocking side to side.

Seven ligaments strap the knee in place: five circling the joint on the outside, and two crisscrossing inside from front to back. Without these tough, fibrous bands the joint would slip and slide chaotically and painfully. In addition, a heavy tendon stretching down from the quadriceps in the thigh, crossing over the kneecap, or patella, and reattaching at the shinbone, adds muscle power to the joint's stability. When the quads contract, they extend the knee joint, and the power of this contraction is delivered not above the knee but across the face of the joint itself and on to the lower leg, binding the knee more firmly in place. One-third of the knee's stability is maintained by the quads and the hamstrings, which control the joint from the rear with a pair of tendons and keep it from overextending.

A solid-enough joint for most tasks, the knee is nonetheless a frequent victim of certain afflictions and injuries. Arthritis often attacks it, roughening the interior and causing pain and stiffness. Situated as it is between the foot, hips, and upper body, the knee also receives regular and often injurious pounding in the course of jogging or running. But it is contact sports that take the greatest toll on the knee. The meniscus can be torn by a blow or collision or by severe twisting, jamming the cartilage between two bones and grinding it to pieces. Cartilage heals poorly because it has little or no blood supply, and thus surgical removal is often recommended, a process revolutionized in recent years by

arthroscopic surgery. This technique permits surgeons to insert a slender device known as an arthroscope—with a lens, a light source, and a surgical instrument attached—into the knee area to examine the joint and remove damaged fibers without major surgery.

Ligament damage can be serious because ligaments don't have much "give," and once they are torn it takes a long time for them to heal. When torn completely, they have to be sutured together. Much of the strain of most of our athletic activities goes to the medial-collateral and anterior cruciate ligaments—the medial-collateral ligament is on the inner side of the knee, and the anterior cruciate ligament is inside the joint. When an anterior cruciate ligament is torn, knee stability may be severely, sometimes even permanently, compromised.

My approach to both types of injury is a conservative one. Unless you are a professional athlete, there is absolutely no reason to rush into surgery. It's much better to protect and rest the injured joint, wait for the injury to resolve itself, and consider your options. Ideally, the knee should be placed in a posterior cast-shell at a 30-degree angle, which puts the knee's ligaments under minimal stress. Ice should be applied frequently to relieve pain and swelling. With serious ligament sprains, after diagnosis by a physiatrist or orthopedic surgeon, I recommend using crutches for two and possibly three weeks in order to keep your weight completely off the injured knee and give the fibers a chance to heal. If after that time your knee remains very painful, and you still have severe pain when you step down and cannot fully extend the knee, you ought to consult an orthopedic surgeon for possible surgical intervention. In the case of severely sprained ligaments, I also suggest wearing a cast for three to four weeks. And then even with the cast removed, it may be necessary to wear a light brace at night (made from a material called orthoplast), to keep you from redamaging the injured ligaments when you toss and turn in your sleep. Such a brace should be custom-made for the best possible fit.

The point is this: Knee injuries should never be taken lightly, but neither do they necessarily constitute medical emergencies that require immediate surgical intervention. Obtain an expert's diagnosis, use ice to reduce the pain and swelling, protect the damaged area by taking your body weight off it, and take time to consider your options.

There are many surgical techniques of modern sports medicine that do provide quick improvement and therefore are valuable for professional athletes. But are they right for you? It's hard to say, because the long-term effects of these procedures still have to be evaluated. Whenever they are, however, I suspect that many will turn out to be no more beneficial than the more conservative treatments we use now.

What is the best way to protect your knee *before* it's injured? Make sure that your quadriceps and hamstrings are supple and strong. The exercises that follow form a basic but effective program designed to build up and maintain your body's natural support system for the knee. They should be done twice a day for the first few weeks, then once a day, either morning or night. Don't overdo it and strain your muscles. Loosen and then strengthen them gradually. You'll add considerably to your knees' capacity to resist injury and to rebound quickly if unavoidable problems occur. Remember to breathe regularly while exercising, and to relax completely between repetitions so that all tension leaves your muscles.

EXERCISE 1

For this hip flexor stretch, which includes the quadriceps muscle, lie on your back on a bed with your knees bent and your feet over the foot of the bed. Bring one knee up toward your chest and hold it in this position by clasping your hands around the

EXERCISE 1

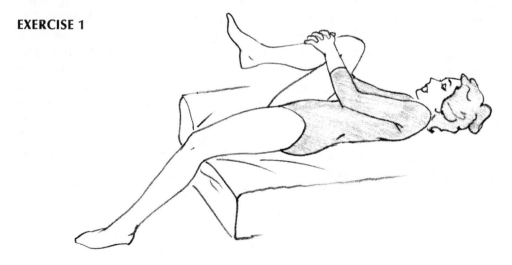

EXERCISE 2

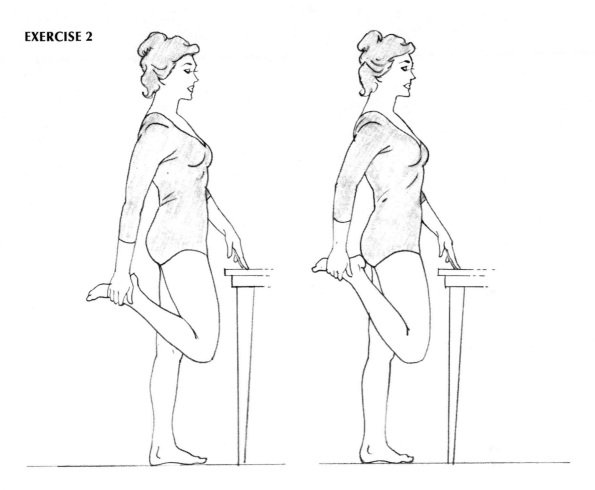

lower leg. Lower the other leg so the knee bends over the edge of the bed and hangs free. Hold this position for 15 to 30 seconds before returning to the starting position. Relax between repetitions until all tension has left the muscles. Do 5 repetitions with each leg.

EXERCISE 2

This exercise is also designed to stretch the quadriceps and hip flexors. In a standing position, and using a table for balance, grab the foot of your injured leg and gently ease your heel up toward your buttock without straining and tilting the pelvis forward. Relax between repetitions until all tension has left the muscles. Start out doing 3 repetitions, holding the stretch for 5 seconds (count to 6). Slowly work your way up to 6 or 7 repetitions, and gradually increase the stretch hold up to 15 seconds (count to 18).

EXERCISE 3

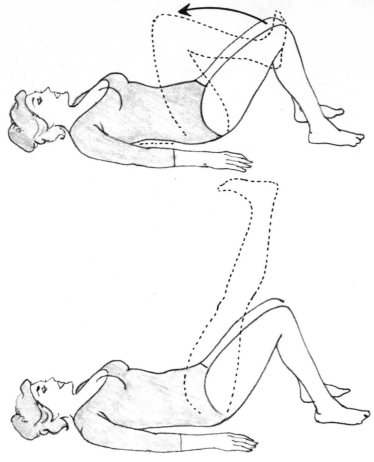

EXERCISE 3

To do this hamstring stretch, lie on your back with your arms relaxed at your side, knees bent, feet slightly apart and flat on the floor. Slowly push the small of your back into the floor while bringing your right knee toward your chest, foot flexed. Straighten the right leg up slowly until the knee is straight. You should feel a pull in the back of your thigh (you may have to lower your straightened leg to achieve this). Hold for 15 seconds (count to 18), then lower your leg altogether and relax for 10 seconds (count to 12). Relax between repetitions until all tension has left the muscles. Work up to 6 repetitions.

EXERCISE 4

If you have any problems with back pain, don't do this exercise. This is another hamstring stretching exercise. Sit on the floor with your legs outstretched before you. Cross your ankles, keeping the side you want to stretch on the bottom. Keeping both ankles relaxed and fully extended, bend forward slowly from the waist, reaching toward your ankles. Do not bounce or jerk your ankles or bend your knees. You should feel the pull on the underside of your thigh. Hold this position for 15 seconds (count to 18). Relax for 5 seconds (count to 6). Make sure that all tension has left the muscles between repetitions. Do 6 repetitions.

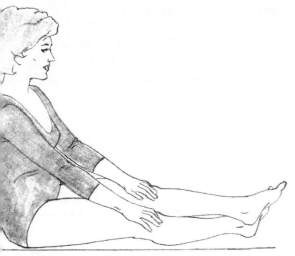

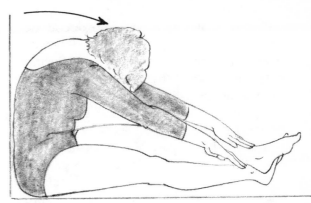

EXERCISE 4

EXERCISE 5

This exercise is designed to strengthen the knee by building up the quadriceps. Lie on your back with your knee bent and your foot flat on the floor. Attach a weight to the ankle of the injured leg which is stretched out with your foot flexed. Press the knee flat on the surface (locking it) and lift the leg to about 45 degrees. Hold it in this position for 5 seconds (count to 6), then bring it down slowly and relax. Make sure that the knee of the injured leg is locked throughout the exercise and that the muscle on the inside of the knee contracts. Start off lifting 1 to 2 pounds 8 times. Gradually build up to 12 repetitions. When these repetitions are easily performed, add another pound and return to 8 repetitions. You may do this until you have reached 15 to 20 pounds.

EXERCISE 5

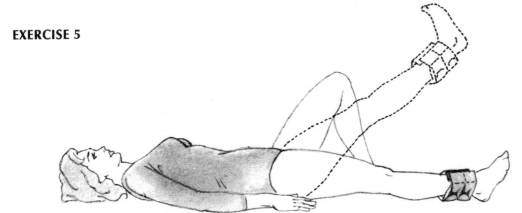

133

EXERCISE 6

This is a flexion-extension exercise designed to strengthen the knee, following the full completion of Exercise 5. Sit in a straight-backed chair with a rolled-up towel or sand-filled stocking under the thigh of your injured knee and a weight attached to that ankle. Flex your foot and raise the lower part of the leg until it is parallel to the floor. Hold for 5 seconds (count to 6), then relax. Start with half the weight that you ended up using in the previous exercise and do 8 repetitions. Gradu-

ally build up to 12 repetitions; once these are easily performed, add another pound and return to 8 repetitions.

EXERCISE 7

This exercise will help strengthen your hamstring muscle. Lie on your stomach with a pillow under your abdomen and a 2-pound weight on your ankle. Slowly bend your knee and raise your lower leg to a 45-degree angle; hold this position for 5 seconds (count to 6), then come down. Another way to do this exercise is to use the full 5 seconds (count to 6) to bend the knee

EXERCISE 6

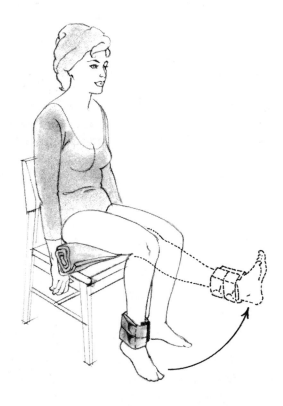

EXERCISE 7

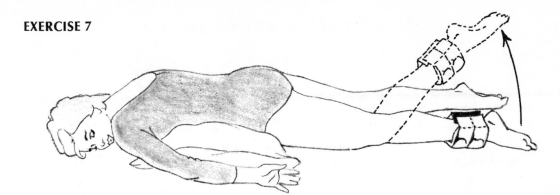

up and down. Be sure to relax all tension in the muscle between each repetition. Start with 1 pound if 2 pounds are too heavy. Gradually work up to 12 repetitions, then add another pound, drop down to 8 repetitions, and work back up to 12.

EXERCISE 8

This exercise is designed to stretch the quadriceps muscle and strengthen the hamstring muscle at the same time. Lie on your stomach with a pillow under your abdomen and a 1- or 2-pound weight on your ankle. Slowly bend the knee beyond a 90-degree angle, then lift the thigh and the calf and hold for 5 seconds (count to 6). Or you can use the full 5 seconds (count to 6) to lift your hip up and down. Gradually work up to 12 repetitions, then add another pound, drop down to 8 repetitions, and work back up to 12.

EXERCISE 5

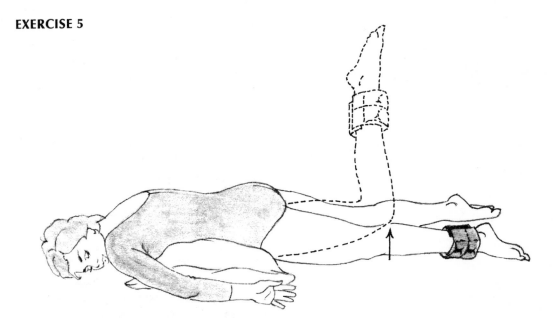

EXERCISE 9

Walk up a flight of stairs, taking 2 steps at once, with your hands behind your back. Without your arms to help balance you, the quadriceps muscle has to do all the work. This is also a good aerobic exercise.

EXERCISE 9

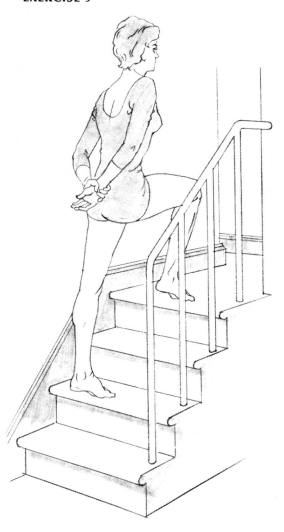

LIGAMENTS

The tough bands of whitish, gristlelike tissue that help bind our joints together are called ligaments. These crucial fibers, which also tightly lace the vertebrae together and assist in keeping internal organs in place, are flexible but not elastic. If severely stretched, a ligament will not return to its normal length and thus may loosen the joint that it secures. If a ligament is extended more than about 5 percent of its length, it may tear or partially rupture, an injury that in extreme cases requires surgery to repair.

Different joints employ ligaments in different ways. The ankle, for example, is held in place by four ligaments: one, called the deltoid, on the inside of the joint, and three on the outside. These outer ligaments are the ones most often stretched in ankle sprains. They are why it is important for your doctor to differentiate between simple ankle sprains (Grade I), in which fibers may be irritated but not stretched, and more serious sprains (Grades II and III), in which stretching or actual separation may occur and joint instability result.

The knee, a largely unstable joint, makes extensive use of ligaments in joining together its basic elements—the thighbone (femur), the kneecap (patella), and the shinbone (tibia). One thick ligament secures the outside of the joint, and two others the inside, while crisscrossing ligaments bind the inner joint surfaces together, running from front to back and vice versa, and provide extra stability. Powerful blows to the outside or inside of the knee can stretch ligaments on the opposite sur-face and even damage the ligaments inside the joint.

Ligamentous injury must not be un-derestimated. If there is a question of such an injury to your ankle or in your knee, I suggest you get a pair of crutches right away to keep any weight off the extremity involved. Then consult a physiatrist or an orthopedic surgeon for advice on further care. In particular, do not take a sprained ankle lightly. There are many active sportsmen whose careers were impaired because of an ankle sprain that was not properly treated. While you may be able to walk on a sprained ankle, there can be a re-sidual instability that sets you up for fur-ther injury, an instability that can also stress the rest of the joint and lead even-tually to the degenerative changes typical of osteoarthritis.

LOW BACK

If you arrive at my office suffering from low back pain, your body is likely to tell me more about your painful predicament than you are, at least at first. This is be-cause you will arrive either with your body twisted like a pretzel from extreme pain, or burdened down with such a heavy load of X-rays and other test results collected from visits you made to other doctors that I might wonder if they are causing your pain! They aren't, of course, but they do reflect the difficulty of evaluating low back pain. Most, but not all, low back problems involve muscle tightness, weakness, and spasm, yet most of the tests usually ordered

by physicians for back pain—including X-rays—are not capable of demonstrating such problems. X-rays show bony struc-tures quite well, but what you see on an X-ray may or may not be related to your pain. Some people have a lot of "findings," or abnormalities, on their X-rays, but they are not in any pain; others may have a lot of pain, but there is nothing on the X-ray to explain it.

An overemphasis on X-ray abnormali-ties of the bony structures in the back has created a number of diagnostic difficulties. Many patients are given what is essentially an X-ray diagnosis, an opinion without benefit of a careful physical examination of the muscles, and without advice about what can be done to correct the person's muscular problems. Some have actually undergone surgery only to discover that it didn't really alleviate their pain, which in all likelihood was muscular in origin.

Not long ago, I received as a patient a woman from abroad who was young and in good condition, but terrified. Suffering from periodic, extremely painful low back attacks, she had been told that spinal fu-sion was the only answer to her problem. Her X-rays showed that the transverse processes, or lateral protrusions emerging from the bony part of the lumbar spine, were slightly enlarged on both sides of the third lumbar vertebra in the low back. Her doctor had concluded that the abnormal size of these protrusions was somehow causing the pain, and that if they could be stabilized by fusion the pain would vanish. It turned out that the patient was a dedi-cated seamstress and often worked long hours standing up and leaning over a large sewing table. This position exerts a great deal of biomechanical stress on all structures of the low back, including the muscles, which in this patient's case responded by frequently going into spasm. The crucial point is that there was no connection between what her X-rays showed and the pain she felt. The enlarged transverse processes were abnormal, yes, but they were not pressing on any structures that could cause so much pain. The pain was being generated by her muscles. Once we determined this, we showed the patient how to work at her table without straining her back and started her on a structured exercise program. She returned home happy and relieved, and well on her way to curing her back problem.

Of course, not all the low back cases we see at the New York Hospital–Cornell Medical Center can be resolved so easily, but while the problem causes more distress to more people than any other except headaches, we have found in most cases that it can be dealt with by strengthening some muscles and loosening others in the system that maintains the trim of the spine. We examine and treat a steady stream of back sufferers in our Department of Rehabilitation Medicine—men and women of all ages and occupations from many parts of the globe—and over the past decade we have been able to help about 85 percent of such patients with carefully prescribed exercise programs and other physical therapy techniques. We also took part in a recent study with the YMCA in which 10,000 back pain sufferers (whose average duration of back pain had been eight years prior to participation in the program) were given some of our therapeutic exercises for six weeks, and 82 percent of them showed substantial improvement. The reason for our success rate is simple: Most of the problems were in the muscles.

In order to understand what we recommend and why we recommend it, you must learn more about the back. It is really a remarkable system, complicated and vulnerable, yet amazingly versatile. Bones, nerves, ligaments, muscles, and tendons are the building blocks of the system. The spine is actually a column that is both flexible and hollow. It is made up of intricately shaped structures, the vertebrae, that are set on top of each other and separated by pairs of gristle-coated, jelly-filled shock absorbers, the disks. There are twenty-four vertebrae and twenty-two disks in the spine, all neatly joined and tightly bound by ligaments. The disks themselves make up 33 percent of the height of the spine.

Inside this armored column, for most of its length, lies the most precious of all cables, the spinal cord, a great bundle of nerve fibers and tissue that links the brain with all the nerves and parts of the body. As the cord descends, pairs of nerves branch out through openings (called foramina) in each vertebra, carrying orders to muscles in the arms, legs, and trunk, and bringing back crucial sensory information.

There are also four sets of muscles involved in keeping the spine constantly upright and taut, like the center pole in a tent or the mast of a ship. One of the more crucial is the abdominal group. Though these muscles don't actually connect with the spine, the abdominals do form a remarkable package of three overlapping layers of crisscrossing fibers that help support the back indirectly. Closest to the surface of the abdomen are the external obliques and the rectus abdominis; these attach to the lower eight ribs and stretch downward to the pelvis. Beneath this outer layer are the internal obliques, which run in the opposite direction, starting at the pelvis and hooking up with the lower ribs. And beneath this second layer lie the transversalis muscles, which run horizontally from side to side and come around from back to front.

The abdominals play a crucial role in keeping your back in line. They help shore it up from the front by assisting the extensor muscles of the back. They also help push internal organs back against the spine by forming a basketlike structure that provides additional support and stability to the lower back. If the abdominal muscles are weak, gravity will drag the contents of the abdominal cavity forward and downward, increasing the natural curve or arch in your lower back. This is an unfavorable situation, requiring other muscles to stretch and tighten in compensation. The back muscles most likely to be thus overstressed are the back extensors, the powerful muscles that run up and down along the spinal column. Their task is to keep the vertebrae well-aligned. The buttock and hip muscles that gird the lower back area may also be affected.

Any structure in the back can cause pain, but in eight cases out of ten, muscles are the villains—muscles that are weak because they are not used, tight because they have gone into spasm, or have lost elasticity from not being adequately stretched.

What is of crucial importance for all potential back sufferers to know is that muscles and muscle tone can be changed without surgery, and usually without medication. The muscles we use for voluntary movement are trainable: They can be made looser or tighter with exercise, and the bony vertebrae of the spinal column they support can be put back into a more favorable alignment and balance.

The typical patient we see at New York Hospital is a person forty years of age or older who is suffering from excruciating muscle spasms in the lower back. Let's assume that it's you: What did you do to deserve this? Well, you probably did very little, including, unfortunately, very little in the way of exercise! But remember, four out of five of us will share this misery at some point in our lives, and it really isn't all our fault. As we grow older, we grow shorter, because the disks in the spine dry out and lose some of their height. This means that the overall distance between the top and bottom attachment sites of our abdominal muscles become slightly shorter and the muscles slacken. In addition, we sit a lot in front of the TV, in cars, in the office, and we tend to do this more as we age. This also creates a slackness in the abdominal muscles.

And so the problem begins: The muscles that flex or bend the hips lose some of their elasticity with the passage of time, and by the age of forty most of us have lost 35 percent of our original hip motion (unless we have been stretching the muscles controlling them). They tighten up so that, as we walk, our pelvis is pulled forward by the hip flexors, delivering excessive stress to the extensor muscles of the mid- and lower back, whose job it is to keep the lumbar spine properly trim and aligned. This is a natural defense against overstressing and overstretching, but it results in painful muscle spasms. Why painful? Because all the fibers in the center, or belly, of the muscle tighten at once. An excruciating cycle is set in motion: contracted fibers have a reduced blood flow, which in turn creates additional pain, and this pain triggers even tighter contractions.

Sometimes muscle spasms do not subside spontaneously and some fibers may remain tangled or clumped. We call such hard muscular knots trigger points, and they are capable of producing a lot of pain. (See Trigger Points). Once they are detected, we inject them with mepivacaine hydrochloride, a local anesthetic, and saline solution that has about the same osmotic, or membrane-passing, pressure as tissue fluid in the human body. The fluid actually pushes the clumped-up fibers apart.

But back to you. You have come to my office twisted like a pretzel, and my first priority is to relieve your pain. First I would have you lie down, and then I'd put an ice pack directly on the area of spasm. Acute low back pain is nearly always caused by spasm of the back muscles, and ice slows transmission time in the pain-conducting nerve fibers. So even though your muscles are still in spasm, you will feel less pain, and this helps break that excruciating cycle. After fifteen to twenty minutes, I would apply some gentle electrical stimulation designed to simulate the contraction and relaxation pattern of normal muscle fibers, another effective way of breaking into the cycle. I might also give you pain medication or muscle relaxants.

Next, I would start you on some low back limbering exercises, designed more to loosen your muscles than to stretch them out. These exercises prevent the muscles from tightening any further and are different from stretching exercises. A muscle in spasm should never be stretched, it would only make the spasm worse. If your abdominal muscles are very weak, I might prescribe some form of back corset.

The two most common tests for low back pain are X-rays and CAT (computerized axial tomography) scans, neither of which provides information about muscle function. CAT scans may show spinal and even disk abnormalities, but they must be interpreted with care, for the changes shown may not in fact be causing you any problems at all. If your difficulties come from nonmuscular causes, however, such testing can be very useful.

Electrodiagnostic studies can also be valuable in cases of "slipped" or ruptured disks, because they can give you an idea of how much actual nerve compression or irritation there is. This test involves putting a very fine needle-like electrode right into the muscles of the legs and back. It may sound painful, but the discomfort should be minimal and well worth the helpful information that can be obtained.

Once I have made your back better with the techniques of my specialty, I would try to protect you against future attacks in two ways. The first would be to give you a specially tailored exercise program, one that you can do at home. After two or three weeks you would then return to the hospital and show me exactly how you are doing your exercises (our records show that very often people are unaware of some little mistakes). I would also give you a booklet of illustrations similar to those printed in this book to remind you how to do the exercises. My second piece of advice would be to find some way of removing yourself from tension. We are all subjected to emotional stress and tension—doctors and medical students, I can assure you, are not excluded. Even should I help make your back better, if you do not come to terms with the sources of your tension, your back may go "out" again. I have my own method, a very simple exercise that children do all the time when they daydream. I pretend to be somewhere else! Remember, as you read what follows, that while we cannot take your tension away, we can improve your resistance against it.

It was some years ago when I learned how to get away from it all without physically doing so. It happened one day when everything seemed to be going wrong. Suddenly I realized that I had to collect my thoughts and establish priorities. So I told everyone to leave me alone, then I locked the door and sat down. For a few moments I wondered what to do. I stared out the window. Then I began to concentrate. I thought very carefully and specifically about hiking up a particular mountain in Austria that I knew well. I thought about the rocks and earth underfoot. I saw and felt the scene in every detail, and I concentrated on each repetitive movement. In a little while I was there on that mountain. My pretend journey was so complete that it had almost become real. I found tranquillity in the familiar and repetitive, and shortly afterward I realized I was ready to go back to work. These days, when the pressures build up, I think about the Norwalk Islands, which are near my home, and I pretend that I am either rowing or swimming there. I perform each physical movement with great care and great concentration. It usually takes me about a minute to get involved, to be "transported," and not more than three or four minutes to complete my pretend journey. I always know when it's time to come home. I feel refreshed and have peace of mind again.

If you feel a back attack coming on, this is what you should do: Immediately lie on your back with your knees bent. Slip an ice pack or cold pack directly under the spot where you felt the tension building. Leave the pack in place for fifteen to twenty minutes, then do the following relaxation exercises while lying on your back: First, inhale through your nose, then exhale slowly and gently through pursed lips (you may do this five or six times); second, gently roll your head from side to side a few times until you feel relaxed; third, bring your shoulders up toward your ears and then let them drop completely. These should then be followed by the limbering exercises at the end of this section (the first three). You may also want to take a couple of mild pain relievers. After about an hour, repeat the ice and exercise sequence.

During the first day you may want to work through this program three or four times, depending on the severity of the attack. In two or three days, the painful muscle spasm should begin to subside. If in the first forty-eight hours your back does not begin to improve, or it gets worse, or you experience a burning sensation when you urinate, you should see a doctor immediately. You could be experiencing the discomfort of a kidney stone or some other medical problem. If pain and spasm do not subside within forty-eight hours, you may need more sophisticated physical therapy

EXERCISE 1

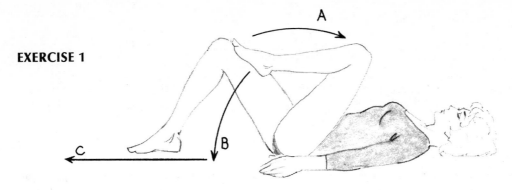

techniques under the guidance of a physiatrist.

No book can pretend to fully diagnose and treat a patient, but it can advise and instruct, and that is how this book can help. But please keep the following points in mind. If you have continuing back problems, and they seem to be exactly like those described in this section, do not try to practice self-diagnosis. Go to your physician of choice. He may refer you to a physiatrist to get a detailed musculoskeletal exam. If you would like to see a physiatrist, but don't know one, you can call a major medical center or hospital and ask for the Department of Rehabilitation Medicine or Physical Medicine. If a specialist in such a clinic feels that muscular problems constitute the main cause of your back pain, then the following exercise program will be of help to you. But please remember: Everybody approaches exercises according to his or her own personality, and thus everybody tends to exercise differently. So, it is extremely important that a qualified specialist, such as a physiatrist, and a physical therapist trained to teach the exercises, design and manage your program—determine how many repetitions you should do, how often, and so forth—and then reevaluate you later to make sure that you are following it correctly. If you are not, it will be of little or no benefit.

In addition to doing the low back exercises that follow, it is also important to read the section "Low Back Body Mechanics."

EXERCISE 1

Lie on your back on an exercise mat with your knees bent and your feet flat. Slowly bring your left knee up toward your chest as far as possible without straining or using your hands, then return your foot to the mat with the knee still bent. Next, slowly slide the heel of your left leg out along the mat until your leg is straight. Gently roll the leg from side to side, then return to the starting position and relax. Exercise your other leg in the same way. Start off doing 3 repetitions with each leg and work up to 6.

EXERCISE 2

Lie on your right side with your knees slightly bent. Place a pillow under your head. Without straining, slowly slide your left knee up toward your chest and lower the knee to the floor. Then, gently straighten out the leg so that your hip and knee are in line with your body, and slightly above your right leg. Finally, drop your left leg onto the right again, so that no effort is used to hold it up. Repeat this exercise three times. Then turn onto your left side and do 3 repetitions with your right leg in the same way; gradually increase to 6 repetitions with each leg.

EXERCISE 2

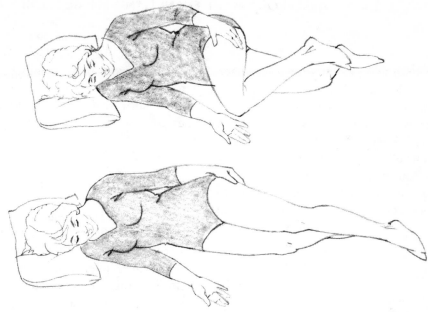

EXERCISE 3

To do this buttocks pinch, lie on your stomach with a pillow under your abdomen. Squeeze your buttocks together tightly, hold for 5 seconds (count to 6), and then relax. Start off with 3 repetitions. If you have difficulty doing this exercise, place one hand on each buttock and gently squeeze them together. Eventually, you will be able to pinch your buttocks together without using your hands. Work up to 6 repetitions.

EXERCISE 3

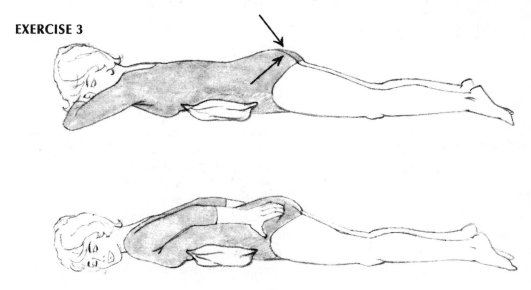

EXERCISE 4

This exercise will stretch your lower back extensors and strengthen your abdominals. Get down on your hands and knees, with your hands directly under your shoulders and your knees shoulder-width apart. Keep your elbows straight throughout the exercise, and make sure your weight is always equally distributed. Stretch by dropping your head, pulling in your stomach while you exhale, and making your back as

round and as high as you can. Hold for 5 seconds (count to 6), then raise your head and relax your back, inhaling as you return to the starting position. Relax for 4 seconds. Start off doing 3 repetitions and work up to 15.

EXERCISE 4

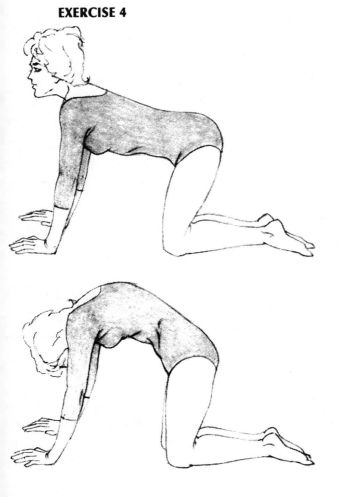

EXERCISE 5

This exercise is designed to stretch your hip flexors. Lie flat on your back with your knees bent and feet flat on the floor. Raise both knees over your chest (see illustration). Bring one knee close to your chest and clasp your hands tightly around the lower leg. Slide your other leg down onto the floor until it is as flat as possible, and try to touch the floor with the back of your knee. Count out loud to 6 while you hold this position, then slowly return to the starting position and relax for 4 seconds before exercising the other leg in the same manner. Start off doing 3 repetitions with each leg and work up to 6.

EXERCISE 6

To do this abdominal strengthening exercise, lie on your back with your arms at your sides. Place a pillow under your knees. While counting to 3, exhale slowly and curl your head forward until your shoulder blades are off the floor. Hold this position for another count of 3, then slowly uncurl with your head reaching the floor last; inhale. Slowly roll your head from side to side and relax. Start off by doing 3 repetitions and gradually work up to 15.

EXERCISE 5

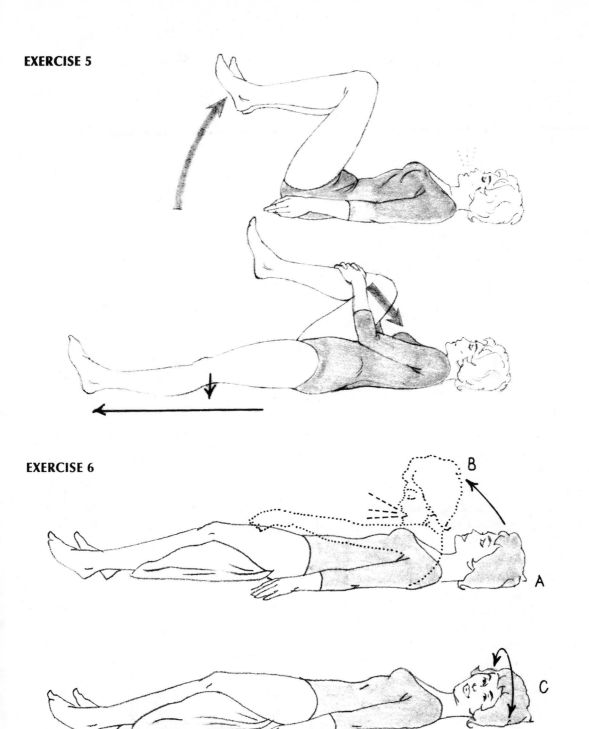

EXERCISE 6

B

A

C

145

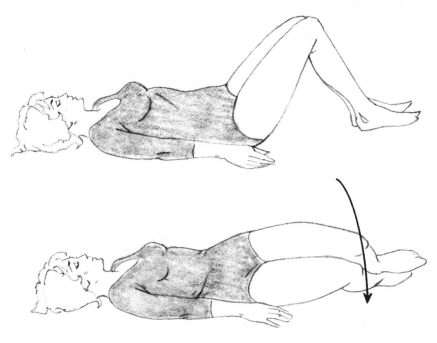

EXERCISE 7

EXERCISE 7

To do this exercise, which stretches the tensor fascia lata muscle, lie on your back with your knees bent, legs together, and feet flat on the floor. Without straining, gently try to lower both knees toward the right side, getting as close to the floor as possible. Do not use any effort to hold your knees on the floor, and do not allow your left shoulder to lift. Hold for 15 seconds (count to 18), then return to the starting position and relax. Lower both knees to your left side. Start off doing 3 repetitions to each side and work up to 6.

EXERCISE 8

To do this upper and lower back extensor stretch, sit in a straight-backed chair with your feet flat on the floor and shoulder-width apart. Let your hands hang loosely at your sides or between your knees. Begin by tucking your chin down toward your chest, then drop your shoulders, bringing them toward your knees. Do not strain or bounce. Hold this position while you count to 6. Tighten your abdominal muscles and squeeze your buttocks together while you return to the starting position by rolling up from your lower back first, then your shoulders, and lastly your head. Relax. Remember to exhale when rolling down and inhale when rolling back up. Start off doing 3 repetitions, and gradually increase to 6.

EXERCISE 8

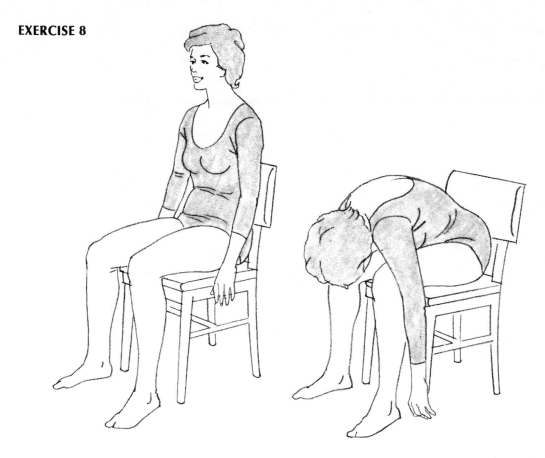

EXERCISE 9

This hip abductor strengthening exercise is done while lying on your side. Lie on your right side, rest your head in your hand as in the illustration. Bend your bottom leg slightly for stability, but keep the top leg straight and in line with your trunk. Slowly raise your left leg as far as you can without straining. Make sure your kneecap faces forward and your leg stays in line with your body throughout the exercise. Count out loud to 6 while holding your leg as high as you can, then lower it slowly, and relax; repeat 3 times. Next, lie on your left side and do the exercise with your right leg. Start off doing 3 repetitions and gradually increase to 12.

EXERCISE 9

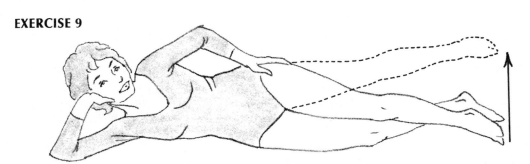

EXERCISE 10

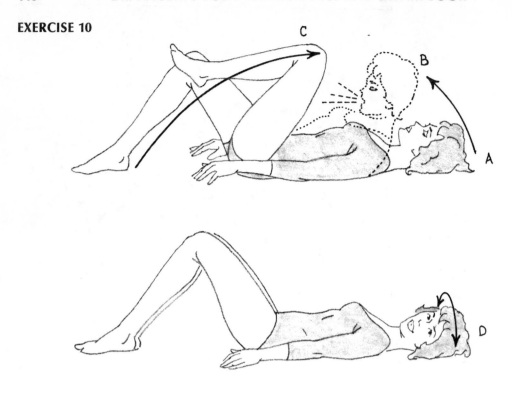

EXERCISE 10

This exercise is designed to strengthen your abdominal muscles. Lie on your back with your knees bent and feet flat on the floor. Keeping your arms at the sides, bring your left knee up toward your chest. Then, to the count of 3, slowly exhale, lift your head bringing your forehead and left knee as close together as possible without straining. Hold this position for another count of 3, then return your head and foot to their starting positions on the floor and roll your head gently from side to side. Inhale and prepare to do the exercise with the right leg. Start off doing 3 repetitions with each leg. Gradually work up to 6 repetitions on each side.

EXERCISE 11

To do this hamstring stretch, sit on the edge of a bed with your right leg outstretched and your left foot on the floor. Flex your right ankle so your toes point to the ceiling, place your hands on your right knee and slowly bend forward, reaching toward your leg with your forehead. (After you make progress, try this with your hands grasping your foot). Keep your right knee straight; do not bounce or jerk. Hold this position to a count of 6 and slowly return to the original position. Exercise your left leg in the same manner. Be sure to rotate your leg from side to side, bend your knee slightly, and relax for 2 seconds between repetitions. Start off doing 3 repeti-

EXERCISE 11

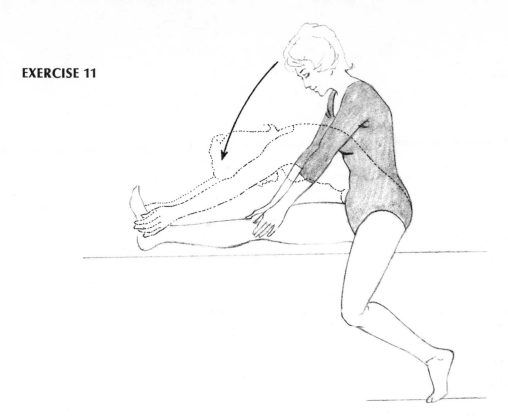

tions with each leg and work up to 6. Exhale while bending forward.

EXERCISE 12

To do this lower back extensor stretch, lie on your back with your knees bent and feet flat on the floor. Lift both knees up toward your chest without using your hands. The small of your back should now be resting on the floor. Gently lower both knees to your right side, and let them rest on the floor for 5 seconds (count to 6). Return your knees to the raised position above your chest and lower them to your left side for 5 seconds (count to 6). Return to the starting position with your knees bent and feet flat on the floor. Relax. Do this exercise 3 times to each side and work up to 6.

EXERCISE 12

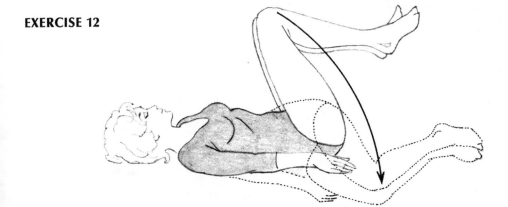

EXERCISE 13

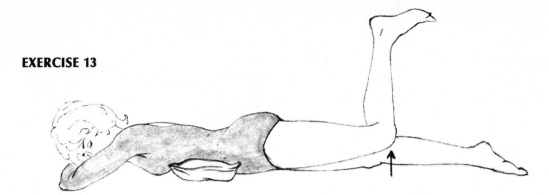

EXERCISE 13

This exercise strengthens your hip extensors. Lie on your stomach with your arms crossed under your head and a pillow under your abdomen. Bend your left knee and raise the leg to a 90-degree angle (the sole of your foot should be facing the ceiling), then raise your left thigh off the floor as far as possible. Try to keep your pelvis flat on the floor. Count out loud to 6, then lower your thigh to the floor. Straighten the knee, gently roll your leg from side to side, and relax. Repeat the exercise with your right leg. Do 3 repetitions with each leg and work up to 10 repetitions.

EXERCISE 14

This exercise stretches your hip abductors. Sit on the floor with your legs outstretched in a V. Bend your knees and move your feet in toward your body until the soles of your feet are together. Grasp your ankles and rest your elbows on the insides of your knees. Press down with your elbows, gently pushing your knees toward the floor. Hold the press for as long as is comfortable, up to 15 seconds (count to 18). Do not force the movement or bounce. Release and relax. Repeat 3 times.

EXERCISE 14

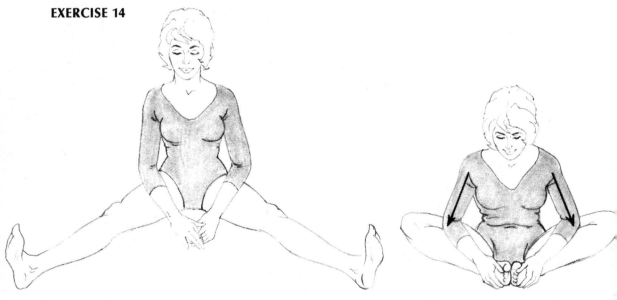

EXERCISE 15

To do this oblique abdominal strengthening exercise, lie on your back with your arms at your sides, knees bent, legs together, and feet flat on the floor. Raise your head and bring your chin down toward your chest. While exhaling, turn your left shoulder toward your right knee. Your left arm should reach beyond your right knee. Lower your left shoulder and then your head to the floor, rest both arms beside you on the mat, slowly roll your head from side to side, and relax. Inhale and do the exercise reaching with your right shoulder and arm toward your left knee. Start off doing 3 repetitions to each side. Gradually work up to 6 repetitions on each side.

EXERCISE 15

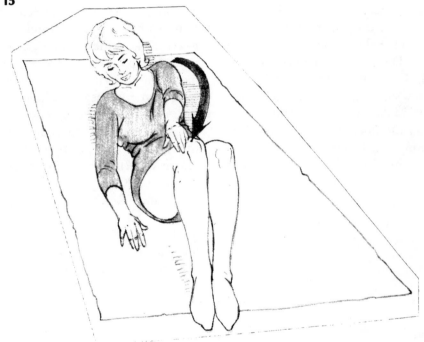

EXERCISE 16

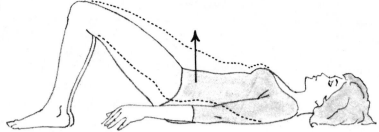

EXERCISE 16

This exercise is designed to strengthen your hip extensors. Lie on your back with your knees bent and slightly apart, and feet flat on the floor. Do *not* place a pillow under your head. Using your upper back and shoulders for support, raise your buttocks off the floor. Make sure your shoulders remain flat on the floor. Hold this position while counting to 6, then slowly lower your buttocks to the floor. Do 3 repetitions, completely relaxing in between and gradually work up to 10.

EXERCISE 17

To do this hamstring stretch, sit on the floor with your legs straight and spread apart in a V. Flex your right foot so that your toes point to the ceiling, place your hands on your right knee, and gently bend over your right leg, reaching toward your knee with your head. (After you make progress, try this with your hands on your foot.) Hold this position for 10 seconds (count to 12), while continually breathing in and out. Keep your knee straight and do not bounce. Return to the starting position, roll your leg from side to side, and relax. Stretch your left leg in the same manner. Start off doing 3 repetitions to each side and increase to 6.

EXERCISE 17

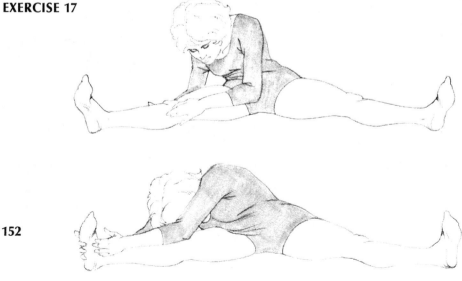

152

EXERCISE 18

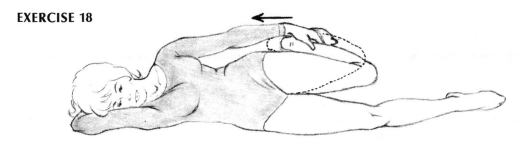

EXERCISE 18

To do this hip flexor stretch, lie on your right side with your head resting on your right arm, keep the right leg slightly bent and behind the left leg. Bring your left heel toward the left buttock; grasp the top of your left ankle with your left hand and pull the knee back past the right leg. To prevent your back from arching, bend slightly forward at the waist. Hold this position for 5 seconds (count to 6) and work up to 15 seconds. Return to the starting position and relax for 3 seconds. Do 3 repetitions with each leg and work slowly up to 6.

EXERCISE 19

This exercise strengthens your back extensors. Lie prone on the floor with two or three pillows placed under your abdomen, and with your arms extended over your head. Simultaneously raise your left arm and right leg so that they are level with the pillows and parallel to the floor. Hold this position for a count of 6, then relax. Repeat the exercise with your right arm and left leg. Start off doing 3 repetitions with each side and work slowly up to 6.

After you have finished with this exercise, you should repeat the first three exercises.

EXERCISE 19

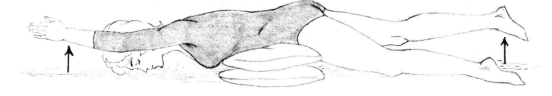

LOW BACK BODY MECHANICS

Very few people get through life without experiencing some form of low back pain. There are two main reasons for this. One is that the area of the lower back is subject to some very powerful mechanical forces and stresses, even during the simplest of daily activities. The other is that—so far, at least—people haven't learned how to protect their backs until *after* they have a problem. Some people suggest that because man is a descendant of four-legged creatures, the human body is unsuited for walking erect. But dogs and horses also have lower back problems, and so that argument should be challenged. If proper body mechanics or back-sparing techniques could be taught early in life—say, to elementary school children—I'm certain a lot of suffering would be prevented. The staggering amount of medical costs and hours lost in the workplace as a result of low back problems would also be reduced. That's why I want to devote a special section to body mechanics for your back. The following suggestions are for *everyone*. Whatever your age, it's never too late to start!

SITTING

At home or at work, sit in a firm chair with a supportive back rest. Try to avoid sitting in very deep or overstuffed chairs or sofas. Doing so may overstretch the back exten-sor muscles that run along the spine, causing them to react by tightening up or going into spasm. Muscles in spasm can be very painful.

When you are sitting in a chair, your knees should be one or two centimeters higher than your hips. This will tilt your pelvis back slightly and relieve some of the mechanical pressures on the lower spine. If you cannot adjust your chair to obtain this position, use a small footstool.

Avoid sitting for long periods; otherwise your muscles may stiffen up and your back be subjected to unnecessary stresses. Get up at least every twenty to thirty minutes and move around, or change positions frequently while you are sitting.

DRIVING

When driving, bring the front seat of your car forward so that your knees are higher than your hips. This reduces the strain on the muscles of the lower back. If the seat is too far from the gas pedal or brake, you will tend to arch your back each time you try to reach the pedal. When your back arches in this way, your pelvis tilts forward; the back extensor muscles, in trying to pull the pelvis back into place, may go into spasm. Also, it is possible to induce a spasm by reaching behind you and yanking an object from the back seat. An inflatable cushion or a contoured pillow can help to forestall back discomfort while you drive.

STANDING

Don't stand in one position for longer than a few minutes. Shift your weight from one foot to the other, or, if the situation allows, put one foot up on some higher object (like a footrail at a bar). When you do this, your pelvis is tilted back and the strain on the back muscles is relieved. If you have to stand a lot, or if you notice low back discomfort whenever you stand for a while, it's a good idea to do daily hip flexor or thigh muscles stretching exercises (see low back exercises 5 and 18 on pages 144 and 153). Tight hip flexors will only tilt the pelvis forward and put stress on the back muscles.

SLEEPING

Sometimes people walk into my office all twisted like a corkscrew from back pain and spasm and quite puzzled by the fact that they were perfectly fine when they went to bed the night before. Certain sleeping positions can trigger back pain and spasm. If you sleep on your back with your arms over your head or behind your neck, the natural curve of your back will increase, stressing the muscles that may then be triggered into spasm. So, if you can sleep only on your back, put a pillow under your knees to relieve some of the stress on the back muscles or try to get used to having your arms at your sides. If you sleep on your stomach, your back will again tend to arch slightly and stress the muscles. If you have to sleep this way, be sure to put a pillow directly under your stomach—that is, at waist level—to flatten out the arch and relieve muscle strain. Probably the best position for sleeping is on your side with your knees brought up toward your chest.

LIFTING

Laboratory studies have shown that lifting heavy objects with your knees bent puts much less pressure on the disks in the vertebral column than if you keep your knees straight. It's also important to hold the object as close to the body as possible. Lifting and arranging something with your arms out and your elbows straight stresses both the upper and lower back. The sequence should be: get close to the object, bend your knees, pick up and hold the object close to your body.

When you go shopping, or come home from work with a heavy load of material, try to divide the burden so you can bear it more or less equally with both arms, thereby balancing the forces on your back.

GARDENING

Before going out to work in the garden, be sure to do some warming up and limbering exercises, just as you would before running or playing tennis. Gardening similarly involves using certain muscle groups repetitively, and often requires bending over for long periods of time.

Keep all the tools you need close by so that you won't have to reach or twist for them. When you are hoeing or raking, keep your knees bent slightly, and stop frequently to stretch. When you reach down for the handles of a loaded wheelbarrow, bend your knees instead of leaning over from the waist and keeping your knees straight. If you weed standing up, don't try to do it by bending over and reaching down to pull the weeds out; loosen them first with a tool, then bend your knees and pull them out gently.

HOUSEWORK

I often see back patients who tell me their pain just came out of nowhere—they weren't jolted by a sudden stop on the subway, they didn't engage in any sports or exercise, and they didn't slip or fall down. On closer questioning, I often find that the pain came a day or two after a dinner party, which took several days of intensive preparation, including vacuuming, polishing, carrying groceries, cleaning windows, lifting stacks of plates. A sudden spurt of increased activity like this places increased loads on the back and greater demands on the muscles, and can often lead to unanticipated problems, especially in someone who is out of shape.

A few suggestions for people who regularly do work around the house: When you are vacuuming, use a handle long enough so that you can stand quite erect and not have to bend over all the time. If you have to move furniture around be sure to push it rather than pull it; this is better for your back. When you set the table, don't reach over to set the opposite side. The same goes for making the bed; walk around to the other side. If you have to reach for an object on a high shelf, use a stool so that you don't have to reach so far and arch your back as much. If the object is heavy, remember to keep your knees bent and hold the object close to the body.

LUMBAR SPINAL STENOSIS

This imposing term refers to a painful lower back (lumbar) condition produced by osteoarthritic narrowing (stenosis) and roughening of the holes (foramina) in your vertebrae through which nerve roots pass. The condition may also relate to a decrease in the diameter of the cavity containing your spinal nerves because of these same changes. If the condition becomes advanced, at certain times and in certain positions bone will press on nerve and you will feel a sharp pain. Osteoporosis, vertebral slippage and collapse, congenital narrowing, and spinal fusion can also contribute to the problem.

Lumbar spinal stenosis is an ailment which we will undoubtedly encounter more often in the future as people tend to live longer. Let's say you come to me and tell me there is nothing wrong with your knees, but you have noticed that walking is not as easy as it used to be. If I examine you and find weakness in the quadriceps, or thigh muscles, on one or both sides, I begin to consider a diagnosis of spinal stenosis. If you are an older patient and I find these weaknesses, you may tell me that when you get up in the morning and stretch, you have shooting pains down your back and legs. If you walk for a while, your calves begin to hurt, but if you sit down, the pain goes away. You can hike up a hill without trouble, but going downhill gives you a lot of back pain. These complaints are different from the ones we hear from patients with bulging or ruptured disks.

What is happening is that the tightness of your muscles, in combination with your body position, are closing off your already narrowed vertebral openings and pressing on the nerve roots. When you sit, the openings become slightly enlarged and you feel less pain. When you stand and your hip muscles are too tight, your pelvis tilts forward, narrowing the gaps and increasing nerve root pressure, making you feel pain again. If you walk uphill, leaning forward, the foramina are open, and you are free of pain. When you walk back down, however, you lean back in order to maintain your balance, the openings narrow, and you feel pain again. If you sleep on your stomach, which arches your spine, you may have pain, but putting a pillow beneath your abdomen, which decreases the arch, can ease the pain. Spinal stenosis can also cause pain on both sides of the body (unlike most disk problems), and the pain may involve the spaces between several vertebrae, not just at one level (again, unlike most disk problems).

Diagnosis can be difficult, however, and the pain of spinal stenosis may be erroneously blamed on a number of other conditions, including the aches and pains of old age, sciatica, and peripheral vascular disease. That is why I must listen to you very carefully and examine you in detail. The CAT scan, with its cross-sectional images, is particularly useful in diagnosing spinal stenosis. If, however, the CAT scan interpretation is uncertain, and I am finding it difficult to decide whether you have spinal stenosis or peripheral vascular disease, I would do a treadmill test. But not the kind you may be familiar with in heart examinations. I would have you walk on the treadmill on a level surface first, and then on an incline. If your pain came sooner on the inclined plane, your problem would more likely be in your blood vessels (peripheral vascular disease). Muscles that don't receive as much blood and oxygen as they need become painful, and walking on an incline dramatically increases the calf muscles' demand for these supplies. Diseased vessels are unable to meet this demand. On the other hand, walking on an upward incline can, as we have explained, *relieve* the pain of spinal stenosis.

Still, X-rays, CAT scans, and treadmills cannot tell you how *much* irritation or damage there has been to the nerve. That is why I like to use electrodiagnostic studies, which can give me numerical data on how the nerve is functioning. (See Electrodiagnosis.) These studies are done in two stages. The first is called a nerve conduction velocity study.

An electrical stimulus is applied to the leg, right over the course of the nerve being tested, and the machine measures the nerve's ability to conduct a stimulus, expressed in meters per second. A delay in velocity indicates nerve damage. The second stage is an electromyographic study, which involves inserting very fine needle electrodes into the muscles being tested. Muscles that are supplied by damaged nerves will also be adversely affected, and this will be reflected in the way their patterns of electrical activity show up on a CRT (cathode-ray tube) display screen. People are often frightened at the prospect of undergoing these tests, but afterward are usually surprised at how simple and painless they are. And for the physician, they provide a useful diagnostic tool and monitoring device.

There are situations where a neurosurgeon should be called in immediately—for example, if urinary function is being compromised by pressure on the nerve or nerves that control it. In such a situation you might complain that urination is difficult, or you have the feeling you cannot empty your bladder. An enlarged prostate gland can cause these problems, too, as can a severe bladder infection. So these conditions would have to be ruled out first. A neurosurgeon should also be called in if the pain is excruciating *and* becoming progressively worse despite all attempts to control it, or if the weakness in your legs is progressing rapidly.

Again, I must emphasize that no decision about surgical intervention should be made solely on the basis of radiographic findings or electrodiagnostic tests. The decision should be based on the patient's clinical symptoms. But surgical intervention, when it is necessary, can save you from some very serious problems in the future.

On the basis of my experience with well-documented cases of spinal stenosis in the Department of Rehabilitation Medicine at New York Hospital, I would recommend the following: If there is no absolute need for surgical intervention, you should undergo a structured exercise program, aimed primarily at strengthening the abdominal muscles and stretching the hip flexor muscles and back extensor muscles—that is, the long muscles on either side of the spinal column, especially in the low back, or lumbar area. This does not, of course, change the bony structure of your spine; it does, however, help to tilt the vertebrae in such a way that there is a bit more room for the

nerves to pass through their openings. Your chances of being helped by such a program are in the 70 to 75 percent range, and you have nothing to lose by trying one. If you do, it's a good idea to have a neurologist in the picture to monitor your neurological status closely, and make sure it is not subtly changing for the worse. (Actually, it is possible to get substantially better even if your neurological examination never changes.)

Since spinal stenosis has much in common with other low back problems, people often wonder why we have a special set of exercises for our spinal stenosis patients. There are several reasons. In contrast to "slipped" or ruptured disk disease, spinal stenosis tends to occur later in life. Since it develops slowly over a long period of time, patients may not be bothered enough by pain to go to a physician, but in the meantime they become deconditioned from relative inactivity. Muscle strengthening exercises therefore have to be started at a much lower level than for typical disk patients. In addition, we have noticed that certain specific muscle groups tighten up more frequently in spinal stenosis patients—the hip flexors and the back extensors in particular have to be loosened. Also, the abdominal muscles are usually quite weak, and not just from disuse. With aging we tend to lose some of our height as parts of the spine wear out. The distance between the rib cage and the pelvis decreases, which gradually produces more and more slack in the abdominal muscles. So in older spinal stenosis patients, abdominal strengthening is particularly important. I have seen many patients altogether debilitated with spinal stenosis improve so much that they were able to resume favorite activities they had had to forego—such as bicycling, golf, and hiking (but not jogging; that would be out)—just from abdominal strengthening.

There are several activities that can help you if you have spinal stenosis. Bicycling is excellent because the seat tips your pelvis up and back slightly, thus opening your foramina, and also provides aerobic benefit. Cross-country skiing, or using a home machine that mimics cross-country skiing, can be good if you make sure to keep your hip flexors sufficiently stretched. We also often use the treadmill as a therapeutic aid in spinal stenosis. It assures symmetrical rhythmic walking which, as mentioned, can very effectively help loosen the muscles. By controlling the speed and the incline, we can gradually build up your walking tolerance while also giving you some aerobic benefits. (Keep in mind that, as with many physical therapy treatments, it may be some time before you can appreciate these benefits.)

Three of the five exercises that follow are designed to loosen your hip flexors. This is important because looser hip flexors will permit your pelvis to tip back, and this will improve access, however slightly, to the nerve openings in your vertebrae. The other exercises are for strengthening the abdominal muscles, which will also help tilt the pelvis back and open the foramina. The optimal backward tilt that can be achieved with such measures is about 7 degrees—not very much, but sufficient to make a person feel much more comfortable. You may find some of the exercises easier to do than others. If this is the case, then by all means limit yourself to the easy

ones. In some spinal stenosis patients, the upper back muscles waste away from lack of use. These people may also start walking in a bent forward position. If you notice this happening, be sure to add some postural exercises to your program (see Posture).

I should also mention that in the event you belong to that 25 percent for whom a nonsurgical program does not help, you should see a neuro- or orthopedic surgeon to discuss the advisability and timing of surgery. It is still early enough even if you have been on an exercise program for three or four months. One of our studies showed no direct relationship between the degree of abnormalities—on CAT scans, X-rays, myelograms, and electrodiagnostic studies—and the need for surgical intervention.

Again, as mentioned earlier in this section, the bony changes in spinal stenosis are subtle and slow-growing, and unless you were a surgical candidate in the first place, your symptoms are unlikely to change drastically over a few weeks.

It is probably best to do these exercises twice a day, before breakfast and supper. They should be performed on a rug or exercise mat, and they should not be done stressfully. If you feel pain during or after the exercises, stop immediately, wait a few days, and resume with fewer repetitions. Remember to breathe regularly while doing the exercises, and to relax between repetitions. It may be difficult and somewhat painful to loosen your hip flexors, but if you do so, you really accomplish a lot in both reducing and managing the discomfort of your spinal stenosis.

EXERCISE 1

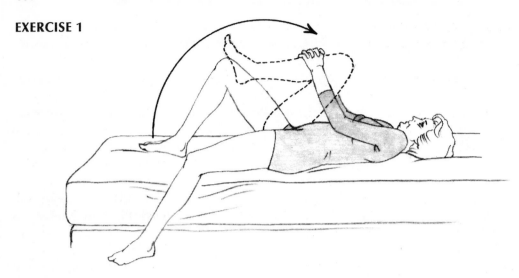

EXERCISE 1

This is a hip flexor stretch. Lie on your back close to the edge of the bed with both knees bent and feet flat on the bed. Bring the inner leg up to your chest and hold it firmly with your hands. Slowly slide the outer leg out straight, then over the side, and let it dangle as illustrated. Hold this position for 15 seconds. Return both legs to the bent-knee position, and relax. Start with 3 repetitions and build up to 6.

EXERCISE 2

To do this hip flexor stretch, lie on your right side with your head resting on your right arm. Keep your right leg slightly bent and behind the left leg. Bring your left heel toward the left buttock; grasp the top of your left ankle with your left hand and pull the knee back past the right leg. To keep your back from arching, bend slightly forward at the waist. Hold this position for 15 seconds (count to 18). Return to the starting position, and relax. Start off doing 3 repetitions with each leg and work up to 6.

EXERCISE 2

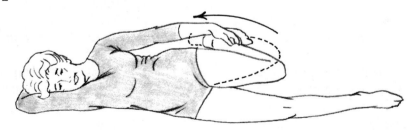

EXERCISE 3

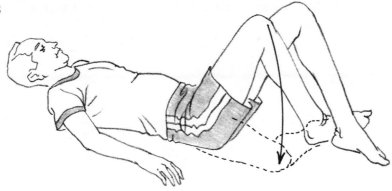

EXERCISE 3

This stretches your inner thigh muscles. Lie on your back with your legs together, knees bent, and feet flat on the floor. Starting with your right leg, hook your right foot behind your left heel. Let the right leg fall gently to the outside without straining. Hold it there for 15 seconds (count to 18). Return to the starting position, relax, and repeat with the left leg. Start off doing 3 repetitions with each leg and work up to 6.

EXERCISE 4

Stretching of the tensor fascia lata muscle, one of the hip muscles, is also important. Lie on your back with arms at your side, legs together, knees bent, and feet flat on the floor. Place the left foot over the right; turn both knees to the right until they touch the floor. Don't strain. Hold for 5 seconds (count to 6), return to starting position, and relax. Do the same thing with the right leg, turning to the left. Do this exercise 3 times to each side. Build up to 6.

EXERCISE 4

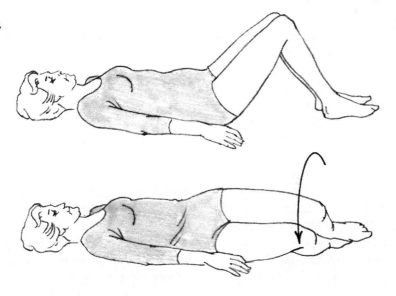

EXERCISE 5

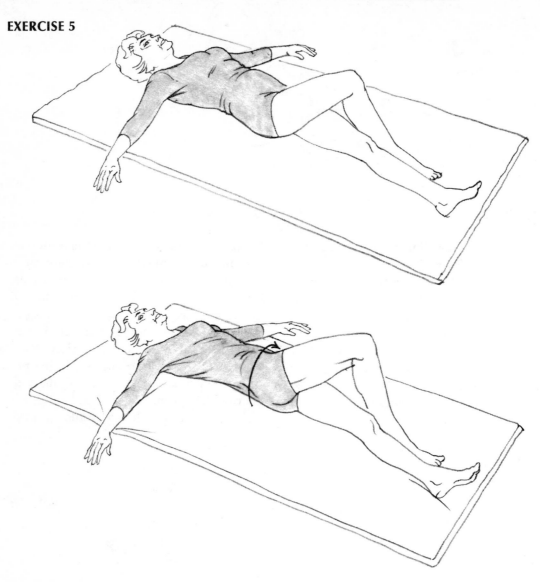

EXERCISE 5

Another hip muscle that often tightens in spinal stenosis is the piriformis muscle. This exercise will stretch it. Lying on your back with both arms stretched out at shoulder height, bring your right foot over the left lower leg, then turn the knee toward the left. Try not to twist; your trunk should stay as flat on the mat as possible. Hold for 5 seconds (count to 6), return to starting position, and relax. Repeat this exercise 3 times on each side. Build up to 6.

EXERCISE 6

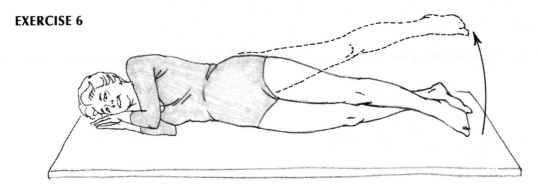

EXERCISE 6

To strengthen the hip abductor muscles, lie on your side with hands under your head and your lower leg slightly bent at the knee. Keeping the upper leg in line with your torso and the knee straight, raise it to about 45 degrees, but no higher. Hold for 5 seconds (count to 6), lower it, and relax. Start off with 8 repetitions and gradually increase to 12. Once this becomes easy, add a 1-pound weight to the raised ankle. Be aware that this is a substantial leverage on the hip, so any increase of weight should be gradual. Turn to the other side and repeat the same regimen.

EXERCISE 7

In order to strengthen the quadriceps muscle, lie on your back with one knee bent and foot flat on the floor. The other leg should be out straight with a 1-pound weight around the ankle. Flex the ankle with the weight so the toes point to the ceiling, tuck in your stomach, tighten the knee, and raise the leg to about 45 degrees. Hold for 5 seconds (count to 6), lower, and relax. Do this at least 5 times. Repeat with the other leg. If you feel any strain in the lower back, do the exercise without weights for about a week, then try again with the weights.

EXERCISE 7

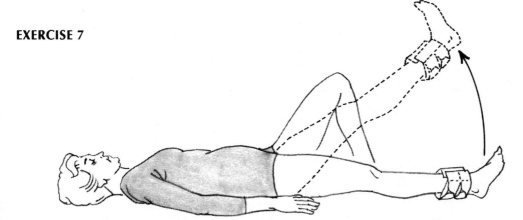

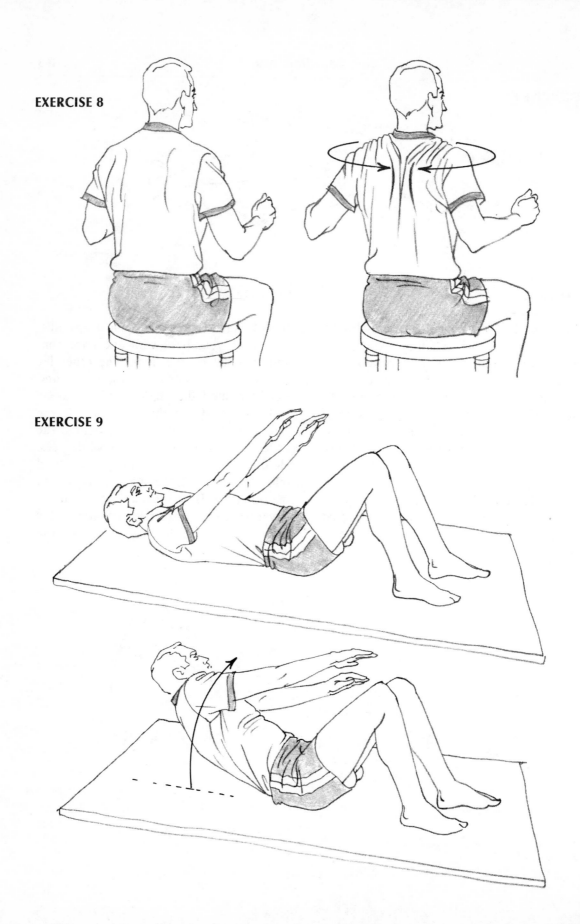

EXERCISE 8

EXERCISE 9

EXERCISE 8

To strengthen the upper back extensors and shoulder blade adductors, sit on a stool, keep your back straight and bend your elbows. Try to bring your shoulder blades together by bringing your elbows and shoulders back. Hold for 5 seconds (count to 6), return to the original position, and relax. Do this exercise 8 times and gradually increase to 12.

EXERCISE 9

Particularly important for the treatment of spinal stenosis are the oblique abdominal muscles. Lie on your back with knees bent and slightly apart, and feet flat on the floor. Stretch your arms forward and come up, reaching with your right hand past your left knee. Return to the original position, then bring your left hand past the right knee. Start off with 5 of these oblique sit-ups on each side, and gradually increase to 10.

Strong abdominal muscles are so important to ease the discomfort of spinal stenosis that I recommend you examine the section on stomach muscles, select the type of sit-up most appropriate to your physical condition, and add this exercise to the above program. As your abdominal muscles become stronger, advance to the next more difficult sit-up.

MASSAGE

One of the most common of all human responses to pain is to rub or stroke the spot that hurts, whatever the cause. Thus it is not surprising that this instinctive response has been expanded over the years into the art and science of massage.

There are various types of massage. Most of them are aimed at loosening up muscles and increasing the circulation or blood flow through the area. As a therapeutic tool, this can be a valuable adjunct to an exercise program. And besides, it usually feels good! Most of the massages given today have their basis in the so-called Swedish school, which teaches several different techniques. One is called the effleurage stroke, which involves gliding the hand over the skin. Petrissage is more of a kneading or squeezing technique. It is very important for a masseur to have a sound foundation of anatomical knowledge in order to judge which technique is best for a particular situation.

Another form of massage, called Shiatsu, which consists of finger-pressure massage over acupuncture points, was recently introduced in this country. True Shiatsu involves a whole philosophical approach to health and healing, but many people use just the pressure point techniques.

There are many other styles of massage, all designed to relax the muscles and increase their blood circulation. Fibrositic massage is used for the muscular condition known as fibrositis. The small subcutaneous nodules that are found in this condition are massaged between the thumb and fingers, and can often be eliminated. Another type is the friction massage, which we use after tendon injuries or tendon repair. Pressure is applied with the thumb in a direction perpendicular to the axis of the tendon. Friction massage seems to have a beneficial effect in preventing the formation of adhesions between tendon and tendon sheath. Follow-up of treatment for tendon injuries does seem to substantiate its effectiveness.

There are some massage devices on the market that claim to provide massaging effects similar to those created by the hands of a masseur, but no machine can take the place of a knowledgeable and skilled masseur. Be wary of heavy vibrating belts sometimes found in health clubs. They will not help you to lose weight and they have no particular value in the treatment of specific musculoskeletal problems.

There are a number of medical conditions that may be made worse with massage. Do not massage your leg if you have phlebitis; massage may break off clots that can then travel to the lungs and create a life-threatening situation. Nor should you massage varicose veins—all it might do is irritate them. Also, it is not a good idea to massage an inflamed joint, such as during a rheumatoid arthritis flare-up, because you might cause the swelling to increase.

Some health centers and health clubs advertise massages for just about any condition. One of them is cellulite massage, which claims to massage fat away. To the best of my medical knowledge, it is impossible for a massage to do this.

The important thing to remember about massage is that it doesn't produce miraculous results or offer any specific healing benefits. I've heard claims that a good Swedish massage has an exercise effect equivalent to a five-mile walk. This just isn't so; the circulatory benefits of massage last no longer than ten or fifteen minutes, and the muscles remain passive throughout the massage. Neither does massage help burn off calories or break down and remove fatty deposits.

Nonetheless, a good massage can relax you, loosen tense or aching muscles, and provide a feeling of well-being. These benefits can be of considerable value, especially if the massage replaces medications, say a tranquillizer. If massage makes you feel comfortable, gets rid of some of your aches and pains, and you can afford it, by all means have a massage!

MUSCLE SPASM

More than 400 voluntary muscles (those that you can control at will) pack the human body to provide the power that makes movement possible. These muscles are composed of tiny fibers—some as thin as thread, some as thick as string—that are bunched together in bundles and contract as a unit, with the individual fibers going in and out of action on a rotating basis during the time the muscle as a whole contracts.

Even when you are sleeping, your muscles continue to contract and relax in order to adjust your body to the particular position you are in.

Sometimes, for a variety of reasons (and sometimes for no detectable reason at all), a particular bundle of muscle fibers will contract instantly and painfully, with all available fibers tightening at the same time. This is known as a muscle spasm. In most cases, you can actually see the contour of the muscle change. Such painful contractions may have modest origins—a cool breeze blowing over tense or overstressed neck muscles, or the failure of one muscle to relax as rapidly as it should during a sudden movement—but they may also be triggered by a painful situation—such as when a piece of ruptured disk in the spine presses on a nerve. When this happens, your muscles "lock" in an effort to form a kind of protective splint so that further irritation will not occur. Unfortunately, the muscle in spasm itself then becomes painful and only aggravates the situation! The muscle fibers contract so tightly that blood flow is curtailed and, consequently, the fibers can't receive oxygen or dispose of waste products. This curtailment of normal functions sets off additional pain signals, and these in turn bring on more contractions.

When a spasm occurs, there are a number of things you can do to help relieve the pain and restore the muscle to normalcy. Some spasms, especially those in the leg, may be mild, and rest, massage, and gentle movement are usually sufficient to break them up. It is easy to get rid of a muscle spasm in the calf by walking—the leg has other muscles, such as the quadriceps and hamstrings, that keep it moving; the calf muscles have to follow along, becoming limbered in the process—but to ease out of a corkscrew position when your back muscles go into spasm may take several days of physical therapy.

Not all kinds of leg cramps are attributable to a muscle spasm. Sometimes the problem is really in the back, especially in the case of lumbar spinal stenosis (see page 156). Older people especially may complain that they get pains in their legs when they are lying on their backs in bed and their legs are stretched out. This position can irritate the nerve roots of the spine by narrowing the openings through which they pass. It's also possible for leg pains to stem from a vascular insufficiency, a compromised blood supply (see the section on Peripheral Vascular Disease). If you have cramping in other muscle groups as well as the legs, you may be having a problem with your metabolism and should consult a physician.

Other muscle groups, especially those in the neck and back, can get caught in a much more vicious cycle, one your body often cannot break on its own. The first and most important thing you can do to break the cycle is to apply a cold pack or ice. This helps in two ways: first, cold dulls the transmission capacities of your pain-conducting nerve fibers, so fewer pain signals will shoot up to your brain, and second, cold reduces fluid build-up in the muscle and thus restricts pressure in the surrounding area, which might be irritating small nerve endings. At New York Hospital, we like to use a third method, especially when the neck and back muscles are involved. This is a special type of electrical stimulation designed to mimic the natural contraction-relaxation pattern of your muscles, thus coaxing them out of their spasm. Anything with the word *electrical* in it may sound drastic, but it's not. The stimulation is very gentle, and patients invariably tell me how good they feel afterward. We then instruct them to move the tight muscle slowly and gently—in other words, to limber it up. This is not the same thing as stretching, which unfortunately is not very helpful for a muscle that is truly in spasm—indeed, it can make things worse.

Limbering helps restore normal circulation and eases your fibers back into their customary patterns of contraction and relaxation.

MUSCLE-TENDON CONNECTION

Tendons and muscles are intimate partners in the remarkable system that moves and powers the human body. Muscles, activated by signals from motor nerves, contract and supply power; tendons, which are tough, fibrous cords with little give, attach muscles to bone and provide muscles with the mechanical leverage to move bone.

The best-known and probably easiest tendon to locate is the Achilles tendon, which runs down the back of the leg from the calf (the gastrocnemius muscle) and attaches to the heel bone. Reach down and grasp the rear of your foot just above the heel. The narrow, ropelike cord you feel is your Achilles tendon. Move your hand up your calf and you'll feel a different texture where the tendon joins the muscle.

In my experience, most muscle ruptures occur at this muscle-tendon junction. It is made of fibers from two different types of tissue, and the combination is more prone to separation than muscle or tendon alone. This is particularly true of the quadriceps and hamstring muscles. The gastrocnemius muscle, however, is an exception. The Achilles tendon, which anchors this muscle in place, is subjected to such stresses that it can become weakened and actually more vulnerable to rupture than the muscle-tendon connection.

A really complete tear at any muscle-tendon junction is rare and usually noticeable. If it happens in the quadriceps, you will know right away—there will be a depression a couple of inches above your knee cap, and you won't be able to extend or straighten your knee at all. If it happens in the hamstrings, you won't be able to feel the hard tendons at the back of the knee, just above and to the side of the crease, and you won't be able to bend your knee when you lie on your stomach.

In the event of a complete tear, surgical intervention is usually advisable. If the tear or "pull" is incomplete, then you can get very good, though slower, results without surgery. Either way, healing occurs with the formation of primitive fibrous tissue to hold the area together again. It usually takes a minimum of six weeks for a muscle and tendon to form a strong new connection. In the early stages of repair, the application of ice packs and gentle limbering exercises are beneficial. Once the connection is restored, the injured muscles have to be strengthened.

MYELOGRAM

When things go wrong with the soft tissues of the body—cartilage, muscles, tendons, nerves, or ligaments—it can be difficult to tell the extent or nature of the damage because X-rays, while effective in depicting damage to bones, are of little value in pinpointing injury or irritation to, say, a nerve being pressed by a spinal disk. A CAT scan may be very helpful in defining the problem or confirming a diagnosis, but if the clinical picture indicates surgery, a myelogram is usually necessary. This is because a myelogram can better pinpoint the location of a disk rupture or fragment, and your surgeon will need to have this information before he operates. The same would hold true if a tumor in the spine were suspected. Unfortunately, a myelogram is an invasive technique, which means that before you take any pictures you have to introduce a needle and some dye directly into the spinal canal. This carries the risk of pain or, at the very least, discomfort during the procedure and for a while afterward, as well as inadvertent damage to neural structures. That is why we recommend a myelogram only when it is quite certain that surgery will have to be performed.

In spite of all the frightful stories about the aftereffects of myelograms (like splitting headaches), I have never encountered a patient who suffered any serious damage from the test. On the other hand, I do not see any reason for a myelogram if a nonsurgical approach is indicated.

NECK AND SHOULDERS

From the first of its seven cervical vertebrae to the last, the neck is an incredibly versatile structure. Unfortunately, it is also a highly vulnerable one.

Consider the tasks this remarkable column of muscle and bone, ligament and nerve must juggle. First and foremost, the neck must be strong enough to hold up the head, which weighs about ten pounds and houses the brain, commander of most bodily functions. In addition, the neck must function as the protector and conduit for the spinal cord, for the eight nerve branches that serve the arms and shoulders, for the pipes that carry food and air into the body, and for four major arteries and veins linking the heart and head.

How can a slender, flexible column do all this? It has to be specially designed for the job. Through millions of years, evolutionary forces have worked and reworked the same mammalian building blocks to create a variety of different but related structures. The giraffe has the same seven cervical vertebrae that you and I have, but in a greatly expanded version, and so does the mouse, which appears to have no neck at all. These vertebrae are separated by disks, covered with a tough fibrous coating, and filled with a jellylike substance.

More than thirty individual muscles ring the neck's vertebrae with guy-wire tautness, enabling the head to move forward and back, to tilt toward the shoulders, and to rotate from side to side for nearly 180 degrees. Not surprisingly in view of such complexity, the neck, head, and shoulders are the target for almost as many painful problems as they have working parts. And when something goes wrong, you know it.

Headaches, neck pain, shoulder pain, back pain, radiating pain, dull aching pain, stabbing pain, numbness, loss of sensation—all can bring you to the doctor's office. Not only that, but the pain felt in the shoulders and neck can come from other locations—the gallbladder, for example, or the pancreas, even the heart. This is known as referred pain. And problems originating in special structures in the blood vessels of the neck can cause high blood pressure and an irregular heartbeat.

External factors can also create neck

problems. Poor posture and overweight, for example, add to the likelihood that you will have difficulties with your neck and shoulders. So does body language, for we speak eloquently with neck, shoulders, and hands, and an excess of such eloquence can create stress and tension in the upper body. Tension in any form, in fact, can tie the neck and its thirty-two finely drawn muscles into knots. Tension causes any muscles to tighten, but the neck muscles, for reasons that aren't entirely understood, are particularly vulnerable in this respect. They also tighten up in response to pain, so if you have a pinched nerve in the neck, your neck muscles will respond by going into spasm. Sitting in front of an air conditioner can cause muscles to knot up, as can sleeping on your stomach, or sleeping with too many pillows or on too soft a mattress. Cleaning windows and painting ceilings can do the job, and so can a tense session in the dentist's chair. Nor are the cause and effect of neck injuries necessarily immediate. Horseback riding, hunting and shooting, and football injuries can all produce osteoarthritic changes in the neck vertebrae that can lead to painful nerve compression as much as twenty years later.

I remember a patient who had severe neck pain because he swam the sidestroke and thus turned his head in only one direction. When he changed to a different stroke, the pain went away. I recall another who experienced pain because his masseur was rubbing his neck muscles the wrong way. When the masseur switched to a form of massage that moved along the length of the fibers, the pain went away.

There is yet another kind of neck stress, one that is usually self-imposed. It stems from extreme exercises and exercise positions, especially those that bend the neck and head back toward the shoulder blades. I know of several cases in which such excessive neck bending from a yoga position or a gymnastic maneuver actually cut off the blood supply in the neck and produced permanent spinal cord damage. In older people, whose cervical vertebrae may already be roughened by osteoarthritis, even modest backward tipping of the head may cause dizziness and fainting. The reasons are the same: When the head is bent backward, osteoarthritic roughening of the vertebrae can temporarily pinch off the arteries that transport blood to the brain.

Diagnosing neck and shoulder pain is a challenge because it is not always easy to sort things out from all these possible causes. One has to approach the problem very logically, beginning wth the patient's story and moving on to a careful and painstaking examination of the muscles, nerves, tendons, and bones. If you were to come to my office, you could expect the following: First, I'd ask a lot of questions. What do you think happened? When did the pain start? Have you had a similar problem before? Have your neck and shoulders been injured, either recently or in the past?

By far the most common problem I see is muscle tightness in the neck and shoulders, often in the form of extremely painful spasms, sometimes accompanied by trigger points, which are hard tangles of muscle. The combination of spasm and trigger points in the neck can cause what are known as cervical (neck) headaches. It is also possible for tight muscles in the shoulder and neck area to cause numbness and weakness in the arm. If I suspect this to be the case, I would have you raise your arm, and move your head from side to side while I took your radial pulse (at the wrist), which would tell me whether changes in the muscle around the neck and shoulders were responsible for reducing blood flow to your arm. If your pulse disappeared temporarily, I'd know that this was the case. I'd also check your reflexes, check for muscle wasting, and check your arms and hands for possible nerve damage.

In all of this I'd use two hands, one guiding the other in my search for trigger points, pressing firmly but gently with the tips of my fingers on your neck. Trigger points in the neck are about the size of grapes, and they are usually found in the "belly," or center, of a muscle. I have to press firmly to find them, and when I do I can feel the knots rolling slightly under my fingertips. Some doctors don't believe in trigger points, but I assure you that they are very real. If you ever develop them you will become a believer, too (especially if I make them go away).

One of my residents had been suffering from headaches for many years. She attributed them mostly to tension and overwork. Aspirin helped, but then she became concerned that she was taking too much. When she started her training with us, she was very skeptical about trigger points, having not heard anything about them in medical school. Since the headache was mostly on the right side of her head, she eventually started to examine her neck by herself, and found a spot that made her headache worse. She came to me for an examination, and indeed I did find a trigger point there. I injected it with a mepivacaine hydrochloride and saline solution and started her on a program of limbering exercises for the neck. Within a few days she happily reported to me that her headaches were gone, and that she could move her neck much more freely than she had in years. I didn't detect any more skepticism—and she gives trigger point injections to her own patients now.

To break up your trigger points, I'd inject a saline fluid that has about the same osmotic, or membrane-passing, pressure as the tissue fluid in your body. Once the injections were given, I'd keep the muscle fibers loose with mild electrical stimulation that mimicked the normal pattern of muscle contraction and relaxation. Your headaches might not vanish overnight, but they would gradually diminish, as they did with our resident, and finally fade away.

You can also develop muscle spasms and trigger points in your shoulder muscles, particularly in the lower parts of the trapezius muscle, the rhomboids, and the paracervical muscles. Though not serious, such tightness can be debilitating, and even though the loss of function may be relatively slight, these muscular problems can develop rapidly. And the time-honored approach of taking X-rays and giving medication is not always helpful. The treatment here, once diagnosis is made, is much more time consuming, though nonetheless effective: a carefully designed exercise program to loosen tight muscles and strengthen those that have become weak.

The next most common neck and shoulder problem I see involves nerve-root pressure. In addition to muscle tension and the bony changes of osteoarthritis, disk wear and tear can produce a bulge or actual rupture of the disk contents. This puts pressure on the nerves, which in turn gives you a radiating pain—unlike that generated by muscle spasms—down into the shoulder and arm. This is known as cervical radiculopathy ("cervical" for neck and "radiculopathy" for injury to the nerve root). Once diagnosed, this pressure may be relieved by the use of traction and therapeutic exercises.

Bicipital tendinitis, frozen shoulder (see page 104), rotator cuff tears (see page 225), and acromio-clavicular (shoulder joint) separations are, in descending order of frequency, the remaining shoulder problems I encounter. The biceps muscles, the powerful two-part unit that fills the front of your upper arm, is attached to the shoulder joint by a thick tendon. This tendon passes through a groove over the head of the upper arm bone. For a number of reasons—perhaps because of overuse, or the loosening of the ligament that holds the tendon in its groove, or a tear in the joint capsule, or calcium deposits—the tendon can become irritated. It may even pop out of its normal position in the groove. Mild cases may be treated with ice applications for twenty minutes at a time, twice a day, and rest. This should solve the problem within a few days. More serious cases should be evaluated by a physiatrist or rheumatologist and may require an injection of cortisone directly into the area of irritation.

The acromio-clavicular joint is situated near the point of the shoulder, where the acromion, the front extension of the scapula, or shoulder blade, meets the end of the clavicle, or collarbone. The degree of separation of this joint is calculated by grade.

Grade I may be treated with ice and rest until it goes away. Grades II and III require specific medical evaluation. Grade II separations may appear less threatening than full separations (Grade III), but if not treated properly they can cause continuing problems. A Grade II separation may require the wearing of a shoulder sling for six to eight weeks, along with an exercise program tailored by your physiatrist to your specific needs.

If you have a full Grade III separation, you may want to consider surgery. If there is no sign at all of nerve injury, exercises for your shoulder muscles could ensure that you would be able to perform all the activities you like, but they wouldn't help you cosmetically—that is, you would still have a permanent bump on your shoulder from the separation. Surgery could improve the appearance, though not necessarily the function. I would definitely recommend surgery if I found some evidence of injury to the brachial plexus, or nerve center for the arms, which would be reflected by neurological changes in your arms or hands.

TENSION-RELIEVING EXERCISES

Of these three exercises, the first is designed to help relieve on-the-job neck and shoulder tension. Some of these exercises may also be helpful in the rehabilitation of specific injuries, but as presented here they are aimed at relieving tension before it causes damage. Remember to breathe regularly while exercising and to relax completely between repetitions.

EXERCISE 1

Sit in a straight-backed chair with your feet flat on the floor and your hands resting in your lap. Slowly raise your shoulders toward your ears, as far as you can without straining, to the count of 6. Take the same amount of time to lower your shoulders to their normal position. Be sure to relax for 4 seconds (count to 5) between each repetition, and concentrate on keeping your fingers and shoulders as loose as possible. Do 6 repetitions of this exercise and work up to a maximum of 12.

EXERCISE 2

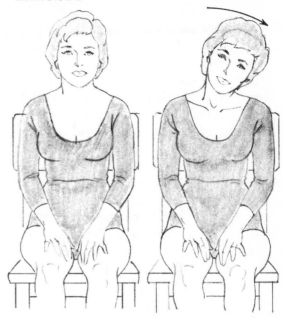

EXERCISE 1

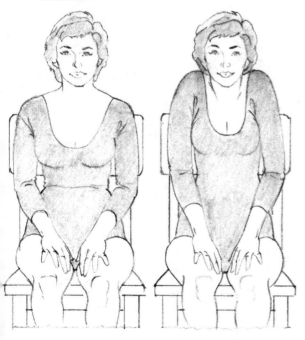

EXERCISE 2

Sit in a straight-backed chair with your feet flat on the floor and your hands resting in your lap. Slowly tilt your head to the left, bringing your ear toward your shoulder as far as it will go without pain. Hold for 5 seconds (count to 6), then slowly bring your head back upright. Repeat the exercise to the right side, hold for 5 seconds (count to 6), then return. Alternate sides until you have completed 6 repetitions on each side and work up to a maximum of 12.

EXERCISE 3

This is a shoulder stretching exercise. Sit in a straight-backed chair, or erect on a stool, with your feet flat on the floor. Raise your arms over and behind your head and firmly grip your right elbow with your left hand. Gently draw your right elbow toward the left side as far as possible without straining. Hold this position for 5 seconds (count to 6), return to the original position and relax for 3 seconds (count to 4). Repeat 6 times, then reverse, grasping your left elbow with your right hand; repeat as above 6 times, working up to a maximum of 12.

STRETCHING EXERCISES

The next three exercises also stretch the neck and shoulder muscles. The first is an excellent shoulder stretch; the other two are designed to be used with applications of cold to relieve muscle spasms, the number-one cause of neck and shoulder pain. When doing these exercises, stretch until you feel the beginnings of a pull. Hold at that point and breathe slowly while the tension eases, then try to go a little further. Do not strain.

EXERCISE 3

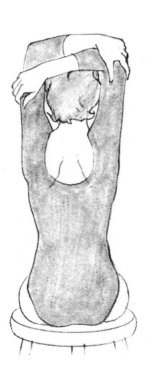
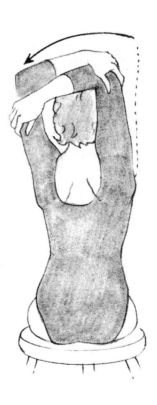

EXERCISE 4

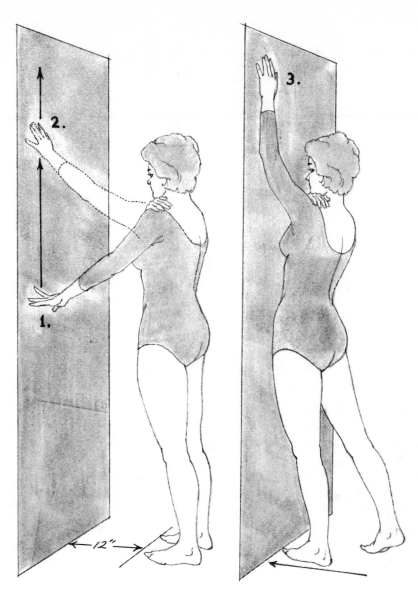

EXERCISE 4

Stand about 12 inches from a wall and raise the affected arm until the fingers touch the wall. Then, pushing down on that shoulder with your other hand, slowly walk the fingers of your outstretched hand up the wall. As you do this, step closer to the wall with the leg on the same side so you can raise your arm as high as possible. Stop when you feel pain. Slowly walk your arm back down the wall, stepping back at the same time. Perform the exercise slowly (count to 6 going up and to 6 coming down), and concentrate on keeping your shoulder down. Start by doing 3 to 4 repetitions, gradually building to 6 or 7.

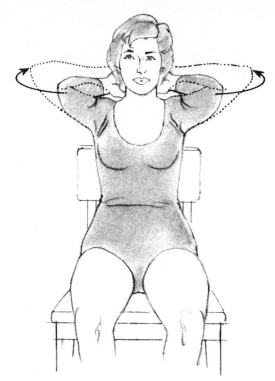

EXERCISE 5

EXERCISE 5

Sit in a straight-backed chair with your feet
flat on the floor, or lie on your back with
your knees bent and feet flat on the floor.
Place both hands behind your neck, then
raise your elbows to shoulder height and
spread them as far apart as possible, gently
forcing them behind you. Hold for 5 seconds (count to 6), return to original position and relax for 4 seconds (count to 5).
Repeat 6 times.

EXERCISE 6

Sit in a straight-backed chair with your
legs together and feet flat on the floor.
Starting with Figure 1 at the bottom of
page 177, move your arms through the different positions: Begin the exercise with
your hands closed, palms down, and arms
straight and crossed at the elbows, right
over left (Figure 1). Open your hands, and
turn your palms up (Figure 2). Then lift

your arms up and over your head (Figure
3). Spread your arms apart (Figure 4).
Close your hands, turning your palms
down (Figure 5). Lower and cross your
arms left arm now over right (Figure 6).
End the exercise with your hands closed,
palms down, and arms straight down and
crossed at the elbows (Figure 7).

Try to move smoothly from one position
to the next and concentrate on the changes
of your hands through the exercise pattern.
Inhale as you open your arms, exhale as
you lower your arms and cross them. Do
this exercise 6 times.

STRENGTHENING EXERCISES

The four exercises that follow are designed
to strengthen your neck and shoulder muscles so that problems will not recur. Build
up your muscles gradually and do not
strain. Breathe regularly while doing these
exercises and remember to relax completely between repetitions.

176

EXERCISE 6

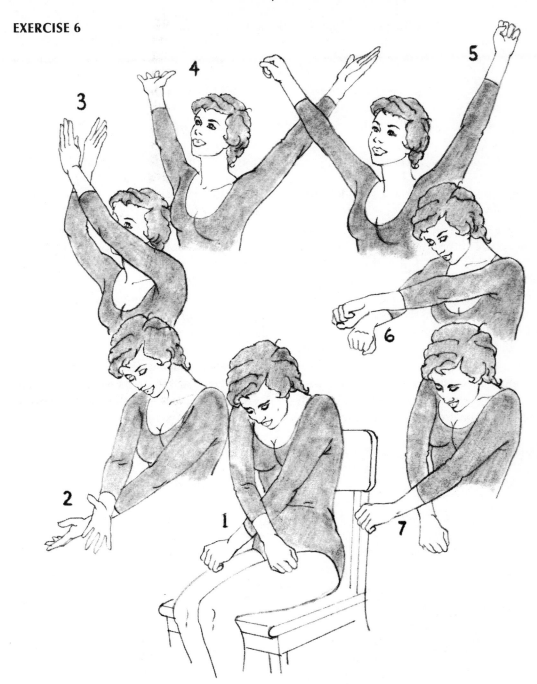

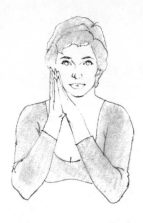
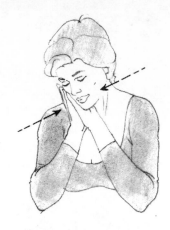

EXERCISE 7

This exercise is designed to strengthen the sterno-cleido-mastoid (neck) muscle. Sit in a straight-backed chair with your feet flat on the floor. Bring your hands together in a praying position and place them on one side of your head. Move your head against the resistance of your hands and hold for 5 seconds (count to 6), then relax until all tension has left your neck muscles. Work the other side of your neck in the same manner. Neck muscles tighten up easily, so you should exercise gently and try to build up muscle strength gradually. Start off doing only 3 or 4 repetitions to each side,

adding another repetition every other day until you reach 15 a day.

EXERCISE 8

Lie on your back on an exercise mat with your knees bent and feet flat on the floor. With a 1-pound weight in your out-stretched right hand, and left arm relaxed at your side, lift your right arm up, keeping the elbow as straight as possible, and slowly, to the count of 6, bring it across your body as far as you can. Then slowly return the right arm to its original position. Relax for 4 seconds (count to 5). Repeat 6 times with each arm.

EXERCISE 8

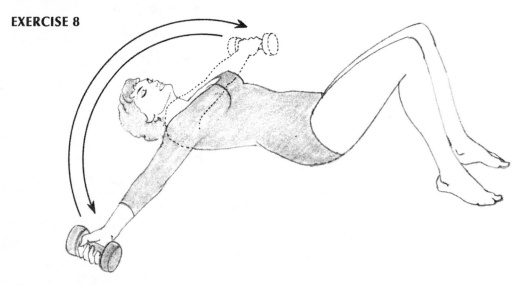

EXERCISE 9

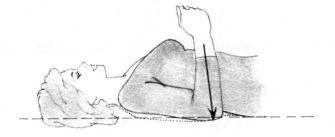

EXERCISE 9

This exercise is designed to strengthen your scapular adductor muscles. Lying on your back on the floor, bend your elbows to a 90-degree angle and push them downward. Begin with 3 repetitions, holding the exercise position for 2 seconds (count to 3), and relaxing between repetitions. Gradually build to 15 repetitions, and to holding each one for 5 seconds (count to 6).

EXERCISE 10

Here is another exercise designed to strengthen the shoulders. Lie on your back with your knees bent, feet flat on the floor and slightly apart, and weights in each hand. Keeping your arms straight and parallel, slowly bring the weights up over your head and down to the floor behind you. Then reverse the direction, bringing the weights back to the starting position. Take 5 seconds (count to 6) to move in each direction. Relax, and repeat.

Use a weight you can comfortably lift in this manner 10 or 12 times—1 or 2 pounds should be sufficient. As you get stronger, add a pound, drop down to 8 repetitions, and work back up to 12. Your goal: to increase to 10 pounds for 12 repetitions.

EXERCISE 10

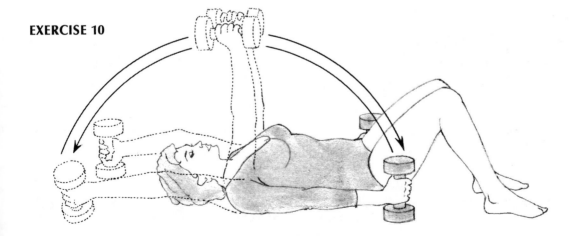

NUMBNESS AND TINGLING

A feeling of numbness and tingling in the face, arms, or legs is a common occurrence as we get older, yet it can be very worrisome to the person experiencing it. In most instances, however, this numbness and tingling is not, per se, a major danger signal. Any kind of pressure on a peripheral nerve—that is, a nerve that goes out to your arms or legs, to your "periphery"—can cause the symptoms. If you can figure out the position in which you experienced it—such as keeping your elbow on a table or crossing your legs—the only treatment really necessary is to avoid that position; the numbness and tingling will spontaneously subside. If you are working at a job that frequently brings on numbness in your hands or your feet, try to avoid the position that causes it; frequent pressure on the nerves could eventually cause permanent damage.

If you have these sensations running down one arm, and don't know exactly why, then you are most likely experiencing pressure on a nerve root in the neck—that is, a nerve in the neck has been pinched by a bulging disk or an osteoarthritic spur. The same thing can happen in the lumbar area of the spine, with these strange feelings radiating into the leg and foot. Either way, it is wise to see your physician, who will probably refer you to a physiatrist or a neurologist. In most instances, the situation can be reversed or improved with a good rehabilitation program, and without surgical intervention.

Sometimes numbness and tingling are accompanied by a feeling of coldness in the affected area. If it doesn't actually feel colder to the touch, then you can be quite sure that pressure on a nerve is the cause. If it *does* feel colder to the touch, then you have a bit more cause for concern and should consult a physician as soon as possible. You may have a vascular problem that is impairing your blood circulation.

Numbness of the face or numbness of one side of the body is also a symptom that should bring you to a neurologist as quickly as possible. Such numbness may be a sign of a transient ischemic attack, or TIA, which means that the blood supply to part of your brain has been temporarily interrupted. This can be treated quite successfully with medication or surgery.

If you have persistent numbness in the thumb, index finger, and middle finger, and perhaps partially on the side of the ring finger next to the middle finger, and this numbness increases with certain activities of the wrist, you can be fairly sure that you have a carpal tunnel problem, for which there are many good therapeutic approaches, (see Carpal Tunnel Syndrome).

One cannot always find the cause of numbness even with a very careful clinical examination. Electrodiagnostic studies are of somewhat limited value in elucidating the cause of numbness and tingling because conduction studies on sensory nerves—that is, on the nerves responsible for these unusual sensations—are not as accurate as motor nerve conduction studies. If your physician suspects something in the central nervous system, namely the brain or spinal cord, he probably will do some so-called evoked potential studies, which can detect an interruption in the nerve conduction pathways from the central nervous system to the periphery. The value of these studies has not been altogether established, however, though they can be very useful in certain injuries of the spinal cord. They are usually best done in large medical centers that have a specific laboratory for them.

NUTRITION

At this time, medical science is not yet in a position to give precise, individualized guidelines for every person's nutritional intake. I realize there are many books on the market claiming to do so, and indeed many popular diet books have some delicious recipes in them. But too many of these books are not based on scientific knowledge and careful long-term studies. We know a lot about advising the diabetic patient on his carbohydrate intake, and great strides have been made in learning how to nourish the hospitalized patient who is unable to eat because of an illness. Otherwise, we have a long way to go.

Nevertheless, certain nutritional facts have become quite clear in recent years. Most of us consume too much meat (protein) and too much fat (cholesterol). Protein overloading can damage the kidneys. And the evidence is strong that high blood cholesterol levels increase the risk of vascular disease, heart attacks, and strokes, and that this risk cannot be completely offset by

vigorous exercise. There will always be people who will doubt the importance of cholesterol, but I think it's fair to say that the possible benefits of low cholesterol intake far outweigh the supposed downside risks.

The old concept that a high intake of protein, vitamins, and salt is necessary to achieve maximum levels of performance is no longer accepted. The muscles use sugar and fat, rather than protein, as their major energy sources during exercise. Vitamins are not a source of energy per se, and water, rather than salt, needs to be replaced when you are exercising and perspiring; too much salt can increase the formation of dangerous blood clots. For very intensive physical activity, the carbohydrate portion of your diet needs to be increased.

Former athletes occasionally come to me with a musculoskeletal complaint and I find them quite overweight. Often they ask how this could be when they never increased their food intake significantly. The answer is simple: A high level of aerobic performance turns the body into a very efficient machine capable of making maximal use of its fuel intake. Once the frequency or level of performance begins to decline, however, this very quality starts to have an adverse effect. Nutrients continue to be absorbed very efficiently, but they do not get used up. Instead, they are deposited in fatty tissue. By the same token, muscle mass built up through exercise can also turn into fatty tissue once the muscles are no longer used frequently.

A lot of research is going on to evaluate the role of diet in the development of cancer, but there is little we have been able to establish with certainty regarding any definite cause-and-effect relationships. Nevertheless, several studies have suggested it would be advisable to avoid certain foods or habits. Obesity itself is associated with an increased risk of cancer of the colon, breast, and uterus. A high fat diet, besides its cardiovascular risk, may be a factor in cancers of the colon, breast, and prostate. Smoked foods, and foods cured with salt or nitrites, have been linked with cancers of the stomach and esophagus. Heavy drinkers, especially when they smoke cigarettes or chew tobacco, have a higher risk of developing cancer of the mouth, larynx, or throat.

On the other hand, you may be able to acquire some protection against colon cancer if you eat high-fiber foods, and against cancers of the larynx, esophagus, and lung if you choose foods rich in vitamins A and C. Bran cereals and raw fruits and vegetables are high in fiber content. Carrots, peaches, spinach, and apricots contain vitamin A. Oranges, grapefruit, and peppers are good sources of vitamin C.

We know that people come in different body types—some are thin and lanky, others more muscular and stocky, still others are on the plump side. It is intriguing to speculate that a thorough understanding of the different genetic and metabolic factors involved could lead to specific dietary guidelines for people with specific body types, but here again we don't have nearly enough information yet.

In my practice, I see many people with osteoporosis—"porous" bones that can break easily—whom I urge to seek advice about their calcium intake. As we get older, we tend to ingest less milk and other calcium-containing dairy products. We also tend to exercise less and less; taken together, these two factors contribute to a weakened bone structure. In addition, older people are likely to be taking certain medications on a regular basis that could be interfering with the absorption into the system of calcium and other nutrients. There is a section later in the book on osteoporosis, which goes into these considerations of bone structure more deeply, but here I just want to emphasize the importance of taking in adequate amounts of calcium, especially as you get older.

The best advice I can give on nutrition is to avoid obesity and overindulgence—especially when it comes to protein, fat, and alcohol—and to maintain a balanced diet that includes the four major food groups (proteins, dairy products, fruits/vegetables, and grains); don't underemphasize fresh fruits and vegetables, and foods with a high fiber content; establish regular eating patterns and maintain them daily throughout life; and finally, maintain an adequate calcium intake.

For more specific guidance, seek out nutritional experts in your area or at a nearby hospital, including physicians with special experience in nutritional matters.

OSTEOARTHRITIS, GENERAL

As bones and joints grow old, they undergo various changes, some of which may be serious while others, though they too may incur problems, are simply responding to the aging process. Not all forms of arthritis (experts estimate that there may be a hundred or more different types) qualify for such a benign distinction, but osteoarthritis does. Also known as degenerative arthritis, wear-and-tear arthritis, osteoarthrosis, and degenerative joint disease, osteoarthritis is not only the least fearful form of the disease, it is also the most common. An estimated 40 million Americans suffer from the ailment, with more than 15 million requiring medical care. If you live long enough, you, too, will probably develop some osteoarthritis, or OA as it is often known for short.

Not only is osteoarthritis common, it has a long and well-documented lineage among living creatures. The presence of osteoarthritis has been detected in the fossilized remains of dinosaurs and cavemen and Egyptian mummies. Even rabbits, dogs, horses, and mice show signs of osteoarthritic changes.

In every case the signs are similar and involve a basic defense mechanism in the joints, one that orders up the growth of new bone in the face of trauma, fractures, or the erosion of the smooth cartilage that lines the interior of joints.

Osteoarthritis can be triggered by a variety of factors that deliver trauma to the joint, and the most common result is the natural wearing away of cartilage, especially in the weight-bearing joints—the knees and hips. Cartilage is a slick, ball-bearing material padding the ends of each bone in the joint and allowing for smooth and pain-free movement. When patches of rough bone, or "spurs," are formed, they impede the natural operation of the joint and can make movement very painful. In the spine, also a target of osteoarthritis, the scenario is slightly different. Your spinal disks, which separate the vertebrae, tend to

thin with age. The ligaments that bind the vertebrae together now rub over different bone sites, and this in turn can lead to the development of spurs, though usually less painful ones than those inside the joint because you don't have bone rubbing against bone.

Repeated external trauma—such as the blows delivered by a football helmet, or the recoil of a shotgun, or the pounding that accompanies horseback riding—can also hasten the development of osteoarthritis. Certain types of labor can also produce OA. The term "farmer's hip" refers to an arthritic condition resulting from hours spent trudging behind and lifting a plow over rocky soil. Miners have more spurs in their spines than nonminers—from shoveling and lifting heavy loads. Ballet dancers have more arthritis in their feet than ballroom dancers because they spend so much time standing or landing on them. But even if you do nothing at all, the chances are high that you will develop some osteoarthritis. These figures tell the story: At age thirty there is roughly a 3 percent chance that you will show some X-ray signs of osteoarthritis in your neck and back; at age fifty to fifty-five the number jumps to 60 percent; and at age sixty or older the figure rises to 87 percent.

The connection between the osteoarthritic changes that show up on an X-ray and the pain and discomfort you actually feel is at best tenuous. There are thousands of people walking around with a substantial degree of osteoarthritis who feel nothing at all, while others, with only modest spur development, suffer a great deal. What does it mean? Well, one explanation is that we don't know enough about osteoarthritis and its relationship to musculoskeletal pain. Another is that the condition of your body—the looseness, or tightness of your muscles, for example—can have an enormous impact on the symptoms that are caused by osteoarthritis. What you do and how you do it can also affect your osteoarthritis. For example, if you are a runner used to jogging on grass or dirt roads and you switch to concrete, you may aggravate the osteoarthritic spurs you have and make them extremely painful. By the same token, if you are recently retired and decide to put up a ladder and paint your house and you suddenly tip your head back, roughened bone or bony spurs in your cervical spine may pinch off blood flow to your brain, and you may suddenly lose consciousness and fall. The message is clear enough: If you are sixty or over, assume that you have some osteoarthritis in your knees, hips, and spine, and avoid sudden involvement with new sports, exercise programs, or punishing activities such as running on concrete or painting the kitchen in a day. Ease into new activities, give your body a chance to adjust, and don't subject your musculoskeletal system to sudden and unusual twists and turns.

Whenever your osteoarthritis acts up, if it does, you can often handle the problem yourself. One factor you should remember, however, is that the pain doesn't always appear exactly where your worst osteoarthritis is located. An arthritic hip can make your knee hurt; osteoarthritis in the upper spine can dispatch pain to your chest or arms. This is known as referred pain, and it can be alarming. If you have doubts about any kind of pain or think some other illness or injury may be involved, see your doctor at once.

Sometimes osteoarthritis causes an acute flare-up with severe pain and visible swelling. In such cases, resting the joint and taking aspirin or another nonsteroidal anti-inflammatory medication can be very helpful. Aspirin, up to eight or ten a day, for several days, is one of the most effective and common medications for osteoarthritic pain and morning stiffness, though you must be careful with aspirin if your stomach is sensitive and you have had problems with ulcers, or if you have had any problems with your kidneys. (Remember, if you are an aspirin-taker and have to undergo surgery for some reason, be sure to tell your doctor; aspirin can reduce the speed with which your blood clots and cause serious bleeding problems during surgery.)

It is also important to use a cane or crutch if you have trouble in one hip or knee. A properly measured and cut cane, used on your good side, will not only help you get around, it will absorb about one-fourth of your body weight and itself provide a third balance point, protecting both joint and muscle. It's infinitely better to use a cane or crutch for a week or two than to limp for a month.

If you are overweight, one of the most important things you can do to help your joints is to lose weight. Since OA is a disease primarily of the weight-bearing joints—the knees, lower back, and hips—it makes sense to reduce pressure on those joints. You may also help reduce pain, additional wear and tear, and the creation of new spurs. An OA flare-up should be a signal to start watching your weight.

Pain tends to inhibit movement, which can be particularly damaging in the case of osteoarthritis because the muscles around your joints play such a crucial role in making your joints work. In the knee, a prime OA target, 30 percent of the joint's stability is maintained by the quadriceps and hamstrings in the thigh. If your knee hurts and you avoid moving it, these vital support muscles can waste away rapidly. And it's unlikely that movement, even vigorous movement, will make your osteoarthritis any worse. In the long run, I assure you, it's extremely important to keep your muscles strong, especially those serving the knee. For this reason, I have included a three-exercise program for the knee at the end of this section. Always remember: Limber and strong muscles are a joint's best friend!

Though the knee may be helped by exercise, the hip, a major OA danger zone, is less easily aided because fewer muscles are involved in the function of this ball-and-socket joint. Nevertheless, you will have some relief from your discomfort if you prevent the muscles around the hips from tightening up. And there is some good news for severe cases: the possibility of surgical replacement of the painful joint by the implantation of an artificial hip. Replacement joints for the shoulder, elbow, and knee exist as well, but they are not as successful as hip replacements and I can't recommend them with the same enthusiasm. If you have suffered progressively from an arthritic hip, and if the joint is completely worn down so that bone rubs against bone and nothing can make the pain go away, you ought to find out from an orthopedic surgeon if you qualify as a candidate for replacement. Try to do this at a major medical center, where thousands of such operations have been performed and a full range of replacement devices will be available. Some hospitals have or have access to a computer system that enables the bioengineers to provide an optimal fit for each individual. The risks are small and the results may be dramatically in your favor.

In the spine, OA is most likely to strike low and high—in the lumbar, or low back, region and in the cervical, or neck, area—because most of the spine's movement takes place in these two areas. In the middle, or thoracic, part of the spine, which anchors the rib cage, there is much less opportunity for movement and wear and tear.

The real value of exercises for osteoarthritis is to help your muscles adjust to the changes the condition created in your body biomechanics. In the lumbar area, where pain is often caused by muscle spasm and muscular tightness and weakness, low back exercises can help loosen and strengthen muscles. The same may be done in the neck, but here roughened bone or bony spurs are more likely to press on nerve roots as they pass out through openings in the vertebrae, and this can cause intense radiating pain down your arm and shoulder. A good defensive weapon that works well for the cervical spine, unlike the low back, is traction. If your osteoarthritis is responsible for producing radiating cervical pain, you may be able to ease it by undergoing a series of traction treatments (see Traction), which will add a bit of breathing room to the span of your cervical spine and help reduce the pressure on your nerve root.

Various kinds of exercise can aid in keeping your bones, muscles, ligaments, and cartilage in good condition and help you withstand the pain and discomfort of an osteoarthritic flare-up. Swimming is beneficial and requires no special preparation. If you exercise regularly, and don't suffer from osteoarthritic pain, then jogging, tennis, and bicycling will help firm up your joint-supporting muscles. One should build gradually to any new level of activity in these sports, however, even if one was a regular participant, and it is equally important to warm up well before every session.

The exercise program that follows—which should be reviewed with your doctor before you attempt it to make sure it does not go beyond your individual capacity—is designed to strengthen the muscles that support and move the knee. Do it once a day, starting at a weight that you can handle comfortably, such as two to three pounds for ten to twelve repetitions. Remember to breathe regularly while doing the exercises, and to relax completely between repetitions. Familiarize yourself with the instructions and illustrations. Most exercises fail not because the principle behind them is wrong, but because the exercises were not performed correctly.

EXERCISE 1

This exercise is designed to strengthen the knee of an osteoarthritic leg by building up the quadriceps. Lie on your back, with the nonafflicted knee bent and the foot flat on the floor. Attach a weight to the ankle of the afflicted leg, which is stretched out. Flex the foot so that the toes are pointed to the ceiling and press the knee flat (locking it); slowly lift the leg to about 45 degrees and hold for 5 seconds (count to 6), then slowly lower it and relax. Make sure that the knee remains locked throughout the exercise, and that the muscle just above the kneecap contracts. Start off lifting a ½- to 1-pound weight 8 times. Gradually build up to 12 repetitions; once these are easily performed add another pound and return to 8 repetitions. Try to work up to 12 repetitions with 15 to 20 pounds.

EXERCISE 1

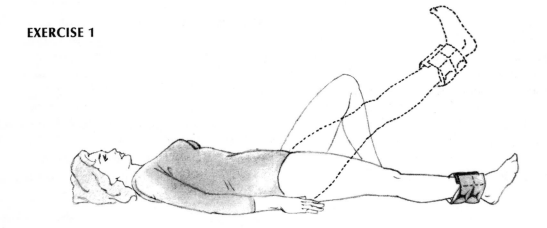

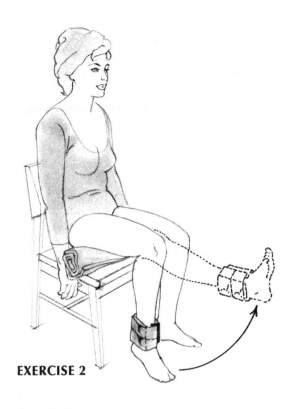

EXERCISE 2

EXERCISE 2

This is a flexion-extension exercise designed to strengthen the knee; it is to be performed after you have strengthened the leg muscles with the preceding exercise. Sit in a straight-backed chair with a rolled-up towel or sand-filled stocking under the thigh on the afflicted side and a weight attached to that ankle. Flex your foot and raise the lower leg until it is parallel to the floor. Hold for 5 seconds (count to 6), then lower and relax. Start with half the weight that you ended up using in the first exer-

cise, and do 8 repetitions. Gradually build up to 12 repetitions; once these are easily performed add another pound and return to 8 repetitions.

If the condition of your knee is extremely painful, you can start off with a 5-pound weight on your leg just below the knee, instead of ankle weights. Although this will build up your quads less efficiently, it's an acceptable alternative. Most people can work this way up to 20 pounds in straight leg raising and 10 pounds in flexion and extension. Do not do this exercise if the pain in your knee increases.

EXERCISE 3

This exercise is designed to stretch your hip flexors. Lie on your back with your knees bent and your feet flat. Bring one knee to your chest and clasp it tightly around the lower leg. Slowly slide the other leg along the floor until it is as flat as possible, then try to touch the floor with the back of your knee. Hold this position for 5 seconds (count to 6). Slowly return to the starting position and relax before exercising the other leg in the same manner. You should feel the stretch in the groin on the side of the straight knee. Do 5 repetitions with each leg, working up to 12.

EXERCISE 3

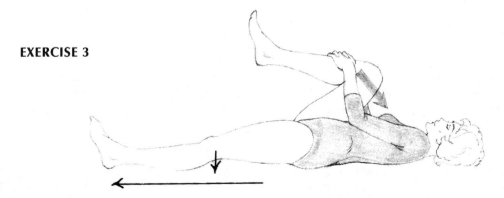

187

EXERCISE 4

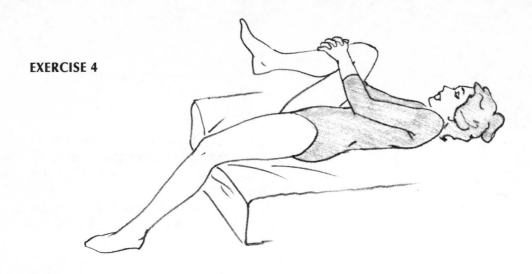

EXERCISE 5

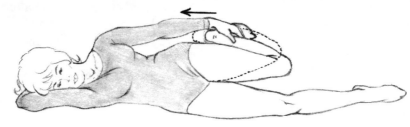

EXERCISE 4

To do this hip flexor stretch, lie on your back near the end of a bed. Bend your knees and place your feet at the edge of the mattress. Bring one knee up toward your chest and hold it in this position by clasping your hands around the lower leg. Lower the other leg so that your knee bends over the edge of the bed and hangs free. Hold this position for 15 to 30 seconds before returning to the starting position. Relax and then repeat with the other leg. Do 5 repetitions with each leg, gradually increasing to 12.

EXERCISE 5

To do this hip flexor stretch, lie on your right side with your head resting on your right arm, keep the right leg slightly bent and behind the left one. Bring your left

heel toward the left buttock; grasp the top of your left ankle with your left hand and pull the knee back past the right leg. To keep your back from arching, bend slightly forward at the waist. Hold this position for 15 seconds (count to 18). Return to the starting position, and relax. Do 5 repetitions with each leg, working up to 12.

OSTEOARTHRITIS OF THE HAND

As explained in the preceding section, osteoarthritis involves degenerative changes in the joints, most commonly those that bear weight, such as the knee and hip. But the hands, given all the work they do, are also affected. Osteoarthritis is much less crippling for the hands than is rheumatoid arthritis, a completely different disease that involves many systems in the body. Osteoarthritis is more related to wear and tear and the long-term effects of injury.

Osteoarthritis of the hand is found more in the finger joints than in the wrist. If you can feel little nodules alongside your finger joints, especially near the fingertips, you probably have osteoarthritis inside the joints. Your hands may be stiff in the mornings, and certain activities, such as opening a jar or a door, can become very difficult. If you find this the case, you should hold your hands in warm water in the morning and do exercises daily. You can't allow your muscles to waste away and stiffen, because the joints will only become that much more painful and restricted. I wouldn't advise you to exercise when you have an acute flare-up, but in the intervals you should do everything you can to maintain the range of motion of your thumb and fingers. The exercises will keep your fingers limber and your muscles strong enough to perform basic skills and daily activities. Just holding a pen exerts a substantial amount of pressure on your finger joints, and the stronger your muscles the better you can handle such everyday situations.

If your hands are severely affected by osteoarthritis, you may need some special adaptive equipment to enhance the function of your hand and diminish the stress on your finger joints. A physiatrist or rheumatologist can refer you to an occupational therapist who can fabricate either a custom-made protective splint or provide special equipment to decrease the mechanical pressure on the joints and enhance the recruitment of muscle fibers.

In some extreme cases it may also be necessary to undergo surgery for joint replacement in the affected fingers, a procedure that requires aftercare by an occupational therapist. Still, every effort should be made to maintain the function of the hand with adaptive equipment, splints, and the help of an occupational therapist.

EXERCISE 1

In order to maintain the web space in your hand—a common problem with osteoarthritis—put both hands together, thumb to thumb and fingertips to fingertips. Try to press the palms together, thus stretching the web space between the thumb and index finger. Hold for 5 seconds (count to 6), then relax. Repeat 5 to 6 times. This exercise should be done daily.

EXERCISE 1

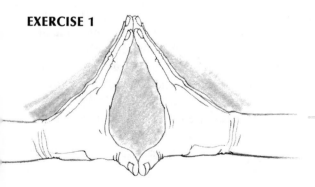

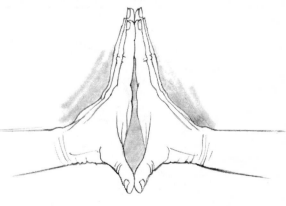

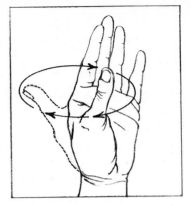

EXERCISE 2

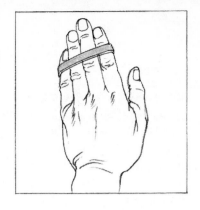

EXERCISE 4

EXERCISE 2

Another exercise aimed at maintaining the web space also improves the mobility of the thumb. Rotate the thumb 5 to 6 times clockwise. Make the circle as large as possible. Repeat 5 to 6 times daily.

EXERCISE 3

To maintain the strength of the thumb muscles, press the thumb of one hand against the thumb of the other hand as shown. Hold 5 seconds (count to 6), then relax. Repeat 8 to 10 times daily.

EXERCISE 4

This exercise strengthens the interossei muscles, which are responsible for spreading your fingers. Wrap a broad rubber band around the fingers as shown, then

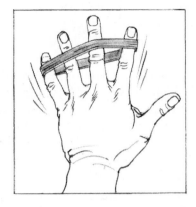

spread the fingers apart. Hold for 5 seconds (count to 6), and relax. Repeat 8 times, working up to 12. Once this becomes easy, use two rubber bands. This exercise should be done daily if you have osteoarthritis of the hand (and skipped on days when you have an acute flare-up).

EXERCISE 3

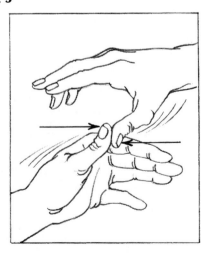

OSTEOPATHY

There are now more than 23,000 osteopaths in all fifty states practicing a medical discipline that differs from traditional, "allopathic" medicine in a number of ways. Modern-day medical practice concentrates on diagnosing specific symptoms and treating them with a variety of therapeutic agents, ranging from medication and surgery to the physiatrist's use of physical methods and the psychiatrist's psychological evaluation and counseling techniques. Osteopathy, on the other hand, takes the approach that if your musculoskeletal alignment is intact, your body's capacity to heal itself will be enhanced regardless of the underlying disease process. Somewhat along the lines of chiropractors, osteopaths are trained in maneuvers and body positioning techniques designed to enhance blood flow and the functioning of the nervous system by correcting misalignments in the spine.

There are numerous, capable osteopathic physicians, and many are particularly skilled in examining and treating the musculoskeletal system. They also play a significant role as general practitioners, as more than 40 percent practice as family physicians in small communities.

In most cases of musculoskeletal pain, in my opinion, it is especially beneficial to the patient to approach problems with means other than systemic medication. I feel that patients will benefit substantially if we encourage and participate in some of the research that osteopaths are now conducting in the biomechanics of the musculoskeletal system. Studies to find ways of preventing musculoskeletal injury by avoiding unusual stress on certain parts of the body in the course of professional labor could save the public money and, more important, decrease the number of work-related injuries or absences from work caused by mechanical stress on certain parts of the body. Such studies and investigations should receive full medical recognition as long as they measure up to accepted scientific methods and principles.

The exception I take to osteopathy is the claim of being able to "adjust" vertebrae. In my opinion, it is impossible to truly do this because vertebrae are tightly bound together by ligaments. Furthermore, ailments attributed by osteopathy to disease-producing misalignments in the spine have been shown to have other causes. The human body can withstand many abnormalities in the spine without any real problems, or even pain. For example, in scoliosis, which is a lateral deviation of the spine, the vertebrae may be "subluxed" or out of position, but many scoliosis patients experience no pain or ill-effect.

Osteopaths receive a basic science education in their own osteopathic schools which is very similar to that found in traditional university-based medical schools. Their entrance selection process is, on the whole, not as rigorous as in traditional medical schools. The clinical training is carried out in hospitals staffed by osteopathic physicians.Their policy for evaluating the merits of their clinical training and therapies is not, in my experience, as open to the same scrutiny as is customary in allopathic medicine. However, I know of many osteopaths whose scholarly attitudes and achievements have my respect.

OSTEOPOROSIS

We tend to think of our bones as solid, unyielding structures—building blocks of careful design and assembly, forming the interior scaffolding that shores us up and ensures movement. Unfortunately, most particularly in regard to osteoporosis, bone is far from unyielding. Like all the body's other cellular structures, our bones undergo constant change, not only when we are young and growing, but also as we become older. The rebuilding process is a kind of biological give-and-take: bones take on some new materials—calcium and other minerals—and at the same time absorb some of the stuff of old bone, roughly in equal proportions. This trade-off is mainly under the control of certain hormones.

It is therefore not surprising that after the hormonal changes of menopause, many women experience an imbalance in the bone-rebuilding equation. Reabsorption of old bone stays about the same, but less calcium and other minerals are taken in. It is almost impossible for women to avoid developing some form of thinning and weakening of their bones. And this deterioration of the skeletal system creates painful and often serious individual health problems. It also adds a heavy burden to the cost of health care in this country, an estimated $2 to $3 billion a year.

Men also undergo a gradual loss of bone density with aging, but since they start off with a higher bone mass and do not undergo the abrupt hormonal changes of menopause, they are unlikely to run into any noticeable problems until their seventies and eighties.

The term "osteoporosis" literally means "porous bones," and it is a condition that makes a person more likely to sustain broken bones—hips, wrists, and legs—after minor falls or collisions. Sometimes the bone actually breaks first and *then* the patient falls! Osteoporotic vertebrae also gradually compress as their inner structure weakens, causing reductions in a person's height, sometimes quite rapid; as much as an inch and a half can be lost for each decade after menopause. Usually the compression is more marked in the front part of the vertebral body, because the downward mechanical forces on the spine are centered there. This is why some women end up with a characteristic rounding of the back and shoulders, known as "dowager's hump." As more and more of the vertebral bodies become wedge-shaped, the spine takes on a curved configuration that can be painful as well as disfiguring. In addition, fragile vertebrae may collapse altogether. Though the bone does not actually make a clean break, the condition is called a compression fracture, and it is quite common in osteoporosis. Compression fractures can cause very painful spasms in the surrounding muscles.

Unfortunately, osteoporosis is not only insidious in its advances, it is also hard to detect. Osteoporotic bone loss does not appear on X-rays until it has reached about 40 percent. A special X-ray apparatus known as a densiometer is a more sensitive technique than chest X-raying for evaluating bone density, especially as a means to check your thoracic spine and detect changes in your vertebrae, but it is not yet widely available.

Ideally, a doctor should also analyze your diet and obtain blood and urinary calcium levels. How much calcium in the diet is enough? The recommended daily amount used to be 800 milligrams, but recent medical research challenged the adequacy of this amount for post-menopausal women, and the generally accepted figure now is 1,500 milligrams—or about three times the average amount consumed by American women older than forty-five. Milk is, of course, a major supplier of calcium—along with yogurt, cheese, other dairy products, dark green leafy vegetables, and sardines—but unfortunately a glass of milk, whole or low fat, provides only about 300 milligrams, and five glasses of milk a day is an unlikely goal for even the most dedicated of calcium consumers, male or female. Thus, calcium supplements make sense, though they may be somewhat less effective than natural calcium in helping the body rebuild its bones. They come in a variety of preparations, of which calcium carbonate has the best chance of being absorbed by your intestines.

Fluorides have not been *proven* beneficial for the prevention or slowing down of osteoporosis, but studies have shown that people who live in areas with fluoride-enriched water have less osteoporosis and fewer dental cavities than the general population. The role of fluorides in the possible prevention of osteoporosis is being investigated.

Many people also feel that hormonal therapy can help retard osteoporotic changes. Those opposed to this approach are concerned about reports that hormonal therapy may increase the risk of certain kinds of cancer. This is an issue that you should discuss carefully with your doctor.

In addition to seeking expert help, there are things that you should know about helping yourself—not to the exclusion of professional guidance, but as a complement to it. First, there are some changes that *only* you can make. Smoking and excessive drinking, for example, reduce your body's capacity to use calcium and other minerals. So, stop smoking and don't drink excessively! Intense and repeated dieting restricts the amount of calcium you get, and too much red meat and coffee can inhibit calcium uptake, as can too little vitamin D.

Perhaps the best news concerning osteoporosis is that exercise can help, especially impact exercises that jar the skeletal structure, however gently. Such exercise retards bone thinning and may even help with the addition of new bone. What happens is that intermittent stresses on the bone create a so-called piezo-electric effect; electrical activity is generated, which in turn stimulates bony growth.

Lack of exercise, on the other hand, increases mineral loss. Astronauts lose 7 percent of the content of their heel bones during ten weightless days in space; nonrunners have a fifth less mineral content in their femurs (the heavy bones in the upper leg) than do distance runners. Six months in bed can drain the bones of nearly 40 percent of their mineral content.

Walking, vigorous dancing, hiking, tennis—all are worthwhile pursuits in the battle against calcium loss. One study of a small number of women past menopause revealed that women who exercised about three hours a week in three hourly sessions added calcium to their bones. Another study, indicated that during a three-year period, women on calcium–vitamin D supplements gained 1.58 percent in mineral content; those on an exercise program added another 2.29 percent; and those in the nonsupplement, nonexercise control group *lost* 3.29 percent.

The implications are clear. If you are concerned about losing bone mass, see your doctor and get his help in planning a program that includes calcium and dietary supplements as well as some form of impact exercise. Swimming, while an excellent aerobic activity and good for keeping your joints moving without placing any stresses on them, does not seem to be as effective as other forms of exercise in curbing the deleterious effects of osteoporosis. Presumably, this is because it puts you in a relatively weightless state where little or no piezo-electric effect can be created.

It is important to keep at your exercise, even if it involves no more than two or three miles of walking three times a week. You will probably gain other benefits as well: you may sleep better, you may be more relaxed, and you may find yourself looking at the world with a more positive attitude.

In general, because of forward curving of the spine and the risk of compression fractures, it is wise to stay away from exercises that involve bending the torso forward. (We do enough of this in our daily activities anyway as we sit at a desk, or reach down into a refrigerator or chest of drawers.) In addition to impact exercise, I recommend the following four exercises, a series designed to counteract the pain and postural problems created by osteoporosis and related muscular inadequacies. It is especially important that they be done slowly and carefully, without undue strain. Follow the order given and then reverse it, so that you work back through from the fourth to the first. They should be done once a day, preferably in the morning, and

it is most important that you do them all. Be sure to breathe regularly during the exercises, and to relax completely between repetitions.

Relaxation inducers should be done lying on your back on a floormat or rug. You should do them with your knees relaxed over one or two pillows. First, inhale through your nose, then exhale slowly and gently through pursed lips (you may do this 5 or 6 times). Second, gently roll your head from side to side a few times until you feel relaxed. Third, bring your shoulders up toward your ears and then let them drop completely. You are now ready to proceed with the exercises.

EXERCISE 1

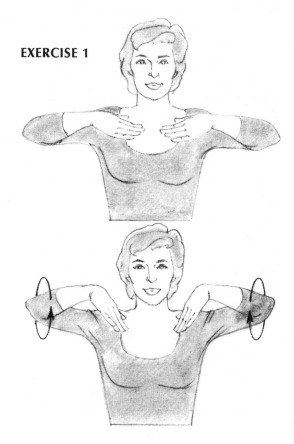

EXERCISE 1

This exercise loosens your upper back muscles. Stand in a relaxed position and place your hands flat just below your collarbone. Pull your shoulders down and lift your elbows to shoulder height. Begin to rotate your elbows clockwise in complete circles, and count the rotations. Do 10 repetitions in a clockwise direction, relax, then do 10 in a counterclockwise direction.

EXERCISE 2

This exercise strengthens your upper back muscles. Lie on your back with your knees bent, feet flat on the floor, legs slightly apart, and place your hands behind your neck with your elbows raised. Lower your elbows to the floor and press them down as hard as you can without straining or hurting yourself. Do not lift your head. Hold this position for 5 seconds (count to 6), then relax. Repeat 10 times.

EXERCISE 3

This exercise strengthens your upper back muscles and stretches the chest muscles. Sit in a straight-backed chair with your feet

EXERCISE 3

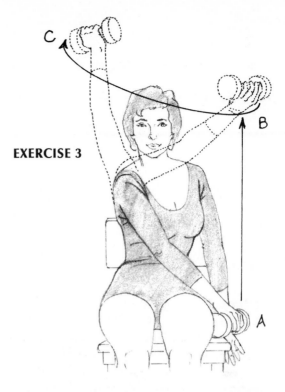

flat on the floor. Hold a 1- or 2-pound weight in your right hand. Place that hand across your body and over your left hip; keep the arm as straight as possible. Lift the weight upward in a direct line from your left hip to your right shoulder. Then, without straining, reach backward. Hold this position for 5 seconds (count to 6), return right arm to left hip and relax. Repeat with the other arm until each arm has performed the exercise 5 times. Gradually increase number of repetitions to 12.

EXERCISE 2

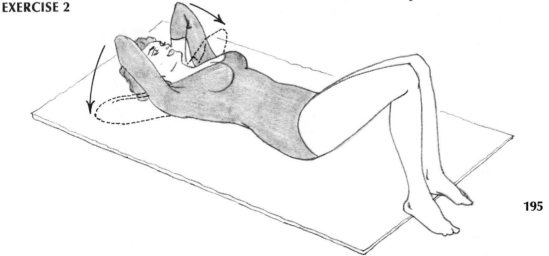

EXERCISE 4

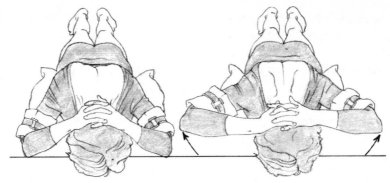

EXERCISE 4

This exercise strengthens your shoulder muscles. Lie face down with a pillow under your waist. With 1-pound weights attached above each elbow, lock your hands behind your neck and lift your elbows as high as you can. Hold this position for 5 seconds (count to 6), then relax for 3 seconds (count to 5). Repeat 8 times.

When you have completed this sequence, reverse the order and work back through all the exercises.

PAIN

We all know what pain is: Something hurts! Yet describing it is difficult. The spectrum of pain may cover anything from the dull aches and sudden, brief pains of daily living to the agony of kidney stones or childbirth. And each one of us experiences pain in a different way, according to our own pain thresholds and our own personality traits. Pain is the primary reason that people take medicine and see doctors all over the world, and it is a complex phenomenon, one that may derive as much of its impact from psychological factors as from physiological ones.

Consider what happens when you hit your finger with a hammer. Metal collides with flesh and a number of chemical substances are released by the damaged tissue, irritating nerve fibers at the impact site. High-speed messages then race up the spinal cord to the thalamus in the brain, a major clearinghouse for pain and other signals, and are finally transmitted into the cerebral cortex. The results: pain perception and response in the form of conscious awareness of what hurts, where it hurts, how much it hurts, and what you say and do about it.

If you are a carpenter long familiar with such accidental collisions, you may simply shake your head and get on with the job. If you are a six-year-old boy who has never been told how to use a hammer, you may cry and run for your mother. To use another situation, if you are in the midst of a football game and someone steps on your finger, you may not feel it at all. Experience, expectation, emotional readiness, even the meaning of the pain itself can have a powerful effect on exactly what you feel.

You may have heard the remarkable

story of the World War II soldier who, when a shell exploded nearby, experienced terrifying pain and felt what he thought was blood dripping down his leg. The soldier, fully expecting to die at any instant, hadn't been hit at all; his canteen had been ripped open, and the fluid he felt was water running down his leg.

Such paradoxes, turning on the constant interplay of mind and body in the perception of pain, make treatment of the problem demanding and difficult. For example, you may come to me for the most fundamental of reasons: You hurt and you need help. But that's just the beginning. The excruciating pain you are experiencing may have started suddenly when you bent over to tie your shoes, in which case it is acute. Such intense discomfort can manifest itself in a variety of ways. There is, however, one particular pattern that you should be aware of and bring to your doctor's attention without delay, and that is *radiating* pain—pain that extends down an arm or leg from its source in the neck or back. This suggests nerve damage or compression, and must be evaluated immediately by your doctor.

My approach to acute pain is very specific. If it is persistent and severe, I will give you enough medication to bring it to a tolerable level. Just how much that should be can get tricky. It is possible to experience side effects from any kind of medication, no matter how little or how much I give you, but if I medicate you inadequately you will continue to suffer, and it will be more difficult for me to examine you and have a good chance of finding out the cause of your pain and what to do about it. On the other hand, I must be very careful not to *over*medicate, because some pain killers are addictive and can cause serious, even life-threatening complications in high doses.

Probably most of us tend to err on the side of undermedicating our acute pain patients. I know of one study that illustrates the problem in convincing detail. It was conducted at a major hospital in an urban setting and showed that more than half of the prescriptions written for severe pain were in fact below the actual dose levels needed to relieve the pain being treated. The reasons for this kind of inadequate treatment varied. In some cases the physicians in charge apparently had some misconceptions about what the optimal dosages actually were; in others, the dosages were not adjusted to keep up with the patient's changing patterns. If a medication is potentially addictive, it is important for the physician to tell the patient all the facts about it, and to make clear that it is being prescribed because it is the best way to bring the patient's suffering under control. If you don't treat acute pain aggressively, you run the risk of turning patients into chronic sufferers.

Pain that has lasted for several weeks or months is *chronic* pain. Again, there is one particular pattern that should alert you to go to the doctor's office, and that is when the pain is persistent and *steadily worsening*. This can be a sign of malignancy or some other progressive condition that should be checked immediately.

The physician's approach to chronic pain (such as may be produced by osteoarthritis, for example) is quite different from his approach to acute pain. Doctor and patient must enter into a longer-term working partnership, one that emphasizes *managing* the pain rather then hurrying to detect and cure its underlying cause. This is not as easy as it sounds, especially if you have been living with your pain for a while. You may become depressed, and such feelings will only reinforce the nagging presence of the pain you feel. In addition, clinical experience suggests that after pain has persisted for several months, specific changes may occur in the nervous system that will echo the pain even if the cause is removed.

This is where your doctor and your partnership with him can help. There are very few true hypochondriacs among those who experience chronic pain, though there are many who may "embrace" their pain and build a life-style around it, one that somehow produces a more influential or satisfying existence. An approach that I find effective in evaluating chronic-pain patients is to ask not about their symptoms but about their *activities* before and after the onset of pain. If the patient finds himself doing less and less of the things he really enjoys, then this may be an indication that his pain is indeed disabling. But if he is following about the same schedule as before, then it's possible the pain may not be as severe as he makes it sound.

Whatever the underlying aspects of chronic pain, doctor and patient must manage it together. To assuage doubts and depression on the part of the patient, I have often found that a structured program, one that is sequential and gradually increases in intensity, can be especially useful in pain management. Whether it involves specific exercises, walking, or even jogging, such a program gives a patient some sense of control and progress, which in turn may induce him to think about things other than his pain. There is no question that those who dwell on pain hurt more, and that those who are active and focus on other things feel pain less. But don't misunderstand me: I don't believe that you can think pain away. What I do believe is that it is possible to become so caught up in other pursuits that you block out some of the painful feelings you have.

Apparently, the body is ready to help in this, if you are prepared to help it with exercise. It is popularly thought that under certain circumstances the brain produces increased amounts of its own pain-dampening chemical substances called endorphins. While it is impossible to say with certainty whether exercise brings about such physiological changes—that is, stimulates the production of endorphins and thereby reduces pain—or whether you feel better simply because you find that you are able to do more than you thought you could, there does seem to be an effect. Perhaps it's a combination of the two!

There is another benefit to regular exercise with regard to chronic pain. If you are active and concentrate on enjoying positive aspects of your life, you may reduce the capacity of pain signals to reach sensory centers of your brain. Research has suggested that only so much sensory information can be processed at any one time by the nervous system. This is known as the gate-control theory of pain, and it is the basis for the success of electrical devices that overload nerve fibers at pain sites in order to *relieve* discomfort. (See TENS.)

The pharmacological industry offers doctors many agents that help him in the management of patients with chronic pain, but this generous supply of medication has its drawbacks. In contrast to the problem of undermedicating an acute pain patient, chronic pain patients risk therapeutic overkill. Unless they engage in a structured therapeutic exercise program, and in as many activities as possible, they may forever remain overmedicated and become an "eternal patient."

Still, one can break into the cycle of pain and depression by using some antidepressant medication for a while, and many pain sufferers respond very favorably to this approach. Of course, the physician alone can also act as an antidepressant agent through his encouragement and guidance.

Perhaps the best advice I can give to any chronic pain sufferer, especially if the pain involves the musculoskeletal system, is this: Don't resign yourself to your pain; make up your mind to fight to be free of it. If you don't know where to turn, I would urge you to seek out a physiatrist, or any other physician who deals frequently with musculoskeletal pain management. I know I may be a bit biased, but a recent market research study did show that some of the most successful results in the management of chronic pain patients are found in major medical centers with well-trained physical therapists working under the close supervision of physiatrists.

PARKINSON'S DISEASE

The cells in our brains communicate in their own special language. Part electrical and part chemical, this mechanism is supremely delicate and subtle, and it depends greatly on having proper amounts of neurotransmitters—chemical substances that help transmit signals from nerve cell to nerve cell, and ultimately to other parts of the body. If this delicate balance is upset, the brain may fail to give just the right instructions, and the person may be unable to perform certain tasks smoothly and naturally.

This is what happens with Parkinson's disease. Dopamine is the name of its crucial neurotransmitter, and for reasons researchers do not yet fully understand, its supply gradually decreases as we grow older. As a result, the brain experiences difficulty in controlling and orchestrating familiar motions. The control system that initiates movement falls "out of sync" with the control system that inhibits movement.

The three major signs associated with Parkinson's disease then begin to appear: tremors, rigidity and muscle stiffness, and hypokinesia, or slowed-down voluntary movement. Not all patients develop all three symptoms, or are affected by them to the same degree, but eventually most suffer from some form of all of them.

Early diagnosis of Parkinson's disease is not easy, for there is no simple laboratory test to help one make it. People afflicted by Parkinson's may become very hesitant in their speaking. They may acquire a stiff, masklike expression, with few wrinkles (causing people around the Parkinson's patient to erroneously assume a lack of emotional reaction.) The first signs of tremor may be slight and appear in only one hand. Whenever the hand is used the tremors will lessen or disappear, and they will not be apparent during sleep, but most any kind of excitement will make them worse. In its early stages, Parkinson's disease tends to rob normal motions of their smoothness and three-dimensional aspect. Patients appear to walk in blocklike fashion, bodies tipped forward, arms stiff, feet shuffling, with little movement in the trunk or hips.

Parkinson's disease affects about 2 percent of all persons over the age of fifty-five, and at present there are nearly a million Parkinson's patients in this country. The figure is increasing by about 50,000 new cases a year. Some neurologists believe that anyone who grows old enough may experience some form of the disease.

Since the early 1970s, a chemical known as L-Dopa has revolutionized the treatment of Parkinson's. This compound helps replace at least part of the missing natural neurotransmitter dopamine, and for a substantial number of those treated the improvement is dramatic. L-Dopa is not a cure, however, for the disease continues to progress even though its symptoms are much less severe.

For this reason, and based on my experience with Parkinson's patients at New York Hospital, I want to offer two important pieces of advice concerning the onset and progression of this disease. First, no matter how dramatic and successful your response may be to medication, you can benefit from a carefully structured exercise program, a program that will help improve every aspect of your daily life. Such a program can also provide you with a sense of doing something on your own to mitigate the disability caused by this progressive condition. Second, if you set your mind to it, you can accomplish an extraordinary range of activities that people around you may have thought you could not do.

I also recommend, if it is possible, that you be treated in a major medical facility by a physician who specializes not only in the care through medication of Parkinson's patients but also in the use of therapeutic exercise programs. I suggest as well that you bring a family member with you, someone who can also learn the exercises and do them with you at home. If you require additional information or guidance, you could contact your state medical board, the nearest university medical center, or the Parkinson Foundation Inc., in New York City.

The exercises that follow are a small sampling of the programs available for Parkinson's patients. I recommend to my own patients that they exercise twice a day, for about a half an hour each time, and then rest for an hour afterward. This rest period is extremely important. Because of lack of synchronization in their muscle-control systems, Parkinson's patients use more energy than the rest of us. They must also be careful to avoid catching colds, and since there is a tendency among Parkinson's patients to feel warm most of the time (because of excessive energy use), they may dress inadequately. Patients also tend to lose weight because they burn so much energy and eat more slowly than normal, often leaving food on their plates when they can't keep up with everyone else.

The point of all exercises should be an increased range of motion in the arms and legs as well as the shoulders and hips. It is also important to keep the muscles of the chest wall as flexible as possible so that the lungs will not be restricted nor breathing affected.

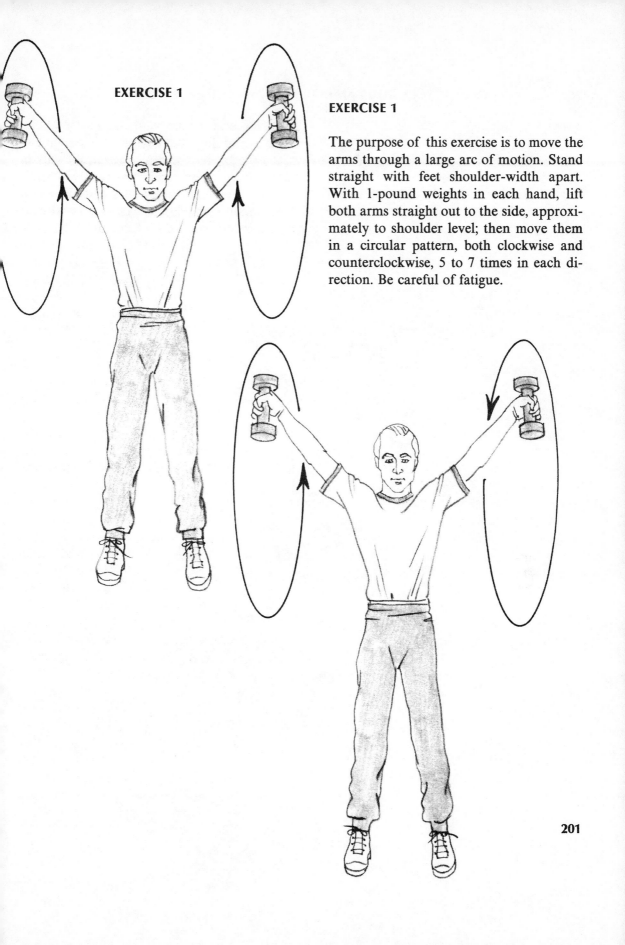

EXERCISE 1

EXERCISE 1

The purpose of this exercise is to move the arms through a large arc of motion. Stand straight with feet shoulder-width apart. With 1-pound weights in each hand, lift both arms straight out to the side, approximately to shoulder level; then move them in a circular pattern, both clockwise and counterclockwise, 5 to 7 times in each direction. Be careful of fatigue.

EXERCISE 2

This is another exercise designed to preserve the ability to move through a large arc of motion. Sit straight on a stool with your feet flat on the floor and arms at your sides. Start with the left arm, bringing it up, over, and behind your head as if you were swimming the backstroke. As you reach the highest point of the stroke with your left arm, start moving your right arm up, over and behind your head (as shown). Do 5 to 10 symmetrical backstrokes with each arm, being careful of fatigue.

EXERCISE 2

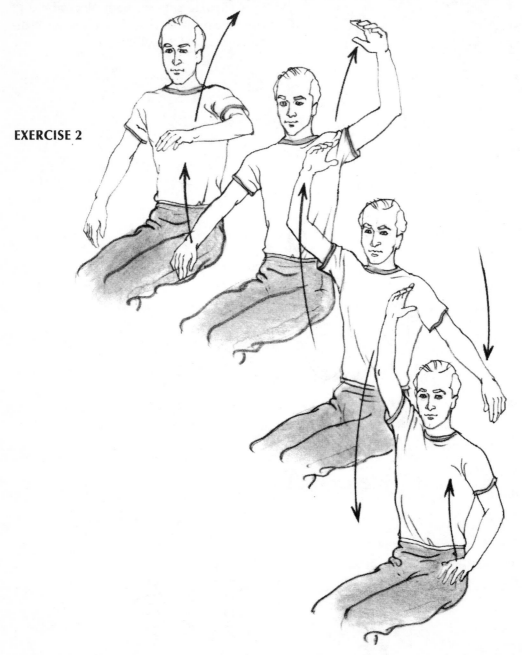

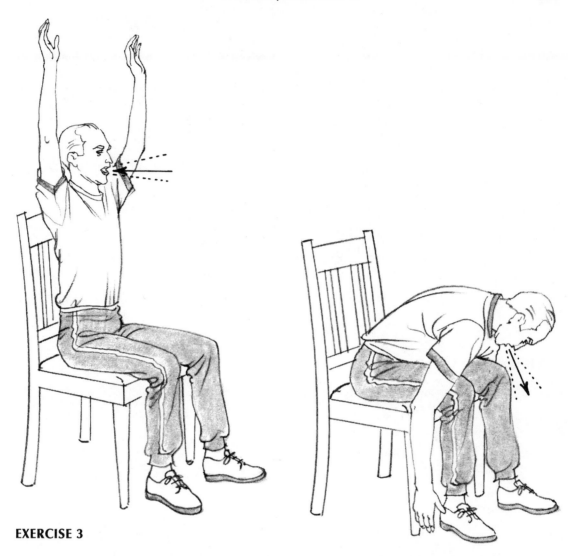

EXERCISE 3

EXERCISE 3

This exercise will help keep your breathing muscles working. Sit in a firm chair with your feet apart and planted firmly on the floor. Take a deep breath as you lift your arms straight up over your head. Then curl forward as far as you can while exhaling. Keep your arms completely loose. Return to upright position. Repeat 8 to 10 times.

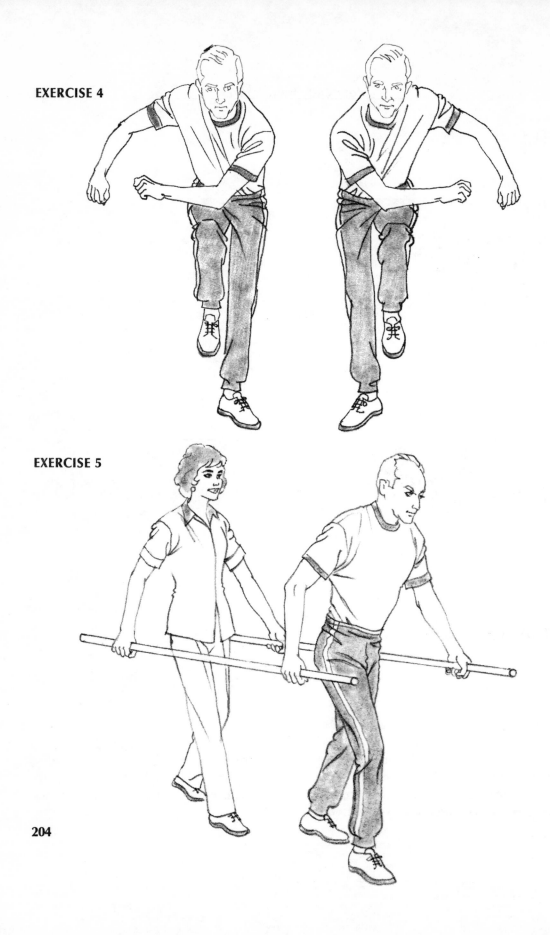

EXERCISE 4

EXERCISE 5

204

EXERCISE 4

This exercise helps you improve the reciprocal motions of arms and legs. While walking briskly, try to bring your left elbow over to your right knee as you lift the right leg, then do the same with the right elbow to the left knee. Exhale as you try to touch elbow to knee. Do this exercise 15 to 20 times.

EXERCISE 5

This exercise works to the same effect with someone else's help. Have another person stand behind you, with both of you holding a pair of poles as shown. In this position you will have to walk in tandem, with the other person's motion reinforcing your own. Make sure that you swing your left leg forward as your right arm moves forward, and vice versa. The person with you must, of course, step and swing the arms in exactly the same manner.

PERIPHERAL VASCULAR DISEASE

The body's veins and arteries form such a sophisticated fluid transport system that even the most brilliant high-tech engineer would have to be impressed. Some blood vessels are thin as hairs, others as thick as your thumb, and all together they are capable of pumping an extraordinary 50 million gallons of blood through the body during an average life span. Yet like most pipes, blood vessels tend to corrode with the passage of time and lose some of their diameter. As a result, blood flow is reduced and oxygen-starved cells in the body's muscles

send out pain signals. When heart muscle cells are involved, the pain is known as angina. When muscle cells in the lower limbs feel pain from such oxygen deprivation, the problem is known as peripheral vascular disease. "Peripheral" means something away from the center of the body—that is, away from the pumping center of the heart; "vascular" is a term referring to blood vessels. So peripheral vascular disease refers to any condition that adversely affects the flow of blood through the extremities, especially the legs.

What happens is this: As blood vessels in the legs narrow and stiffen with age, they lose some of the capacity to expand and contract as oxygen-rich blood is pumped down into them by the heart. The first muscle to respond to such oxygen-reduction is almost always the calf muscle, the gastrocnemius. With its 1,200 muscle fibers per nerve branch (more than any other muscle in the body), the gastrocnemius is extremely sensitive to oxygen loss of any kind. In severe cases of peripheral vascular disease, the results of such oxygen deprivation may lead to gangrene, and ultimately require an amputation. Deposits that form on the inner wall of the arteries can also break loose and form an arterial embolus, which blocks the flow of blood completely. A thrombus, or a clot that develops in one place without breaking loose, can cause the same problem. Either way, gangrene can occur and, again, necessitate an amputation.

This is why it is important to see your doctor when you detect any early warning signs of the disease. Clotting can often be controlled, and in some cases amputation avoided (there are bypass techniques that can be used to maximize circulation in your legs), but early detection is crucial. There are a number of signs you should watch for. One is loss of the little tufts of hair that normally grow on the tops of your toes. If you notice these missing, I recommend that you see your doctor and ask about the state of your arterial circulation. Another more serious sign of encroaching vascular disease is unusual coldness or numbness or pain in your feet. Normally, I'm not all that enthusiastic about diagnostic tests and overdoing it with visits to the doctor, but in the case of this disease I would urge you not to ignore any of these danger signs. I would also suggest in the strongest possible terms that you stop smoking or using tobacco in any form. Smoking even a few cigarettes can send the arteries into spasm, and such blood-vessel constrictions can undermine any and all treatments your doctor may be trying.

One of the reasons that early medical examination is so critical is that other conditions, including arrhythmias (irregular beats) of the heart and spinal stenosis, can produce symptoms very similar to those of peripheral vascular disease.

There are a number of drugs, known as vasodilators, that someone may prescribe to counter the narrowing of the peripheral blood vessels, but exercise, particularly walking, is the best medicine of all. Still, even slow walking can sometimes be painful for the peripheral vascular patient. Exercise bicycles can be easier, though you should understand that as you pedal, blood may concentrate in your quadriceps and hamstrings in the thigh, and not in your lower legs and calf where it's most needed.

To guard against this, raise the seat on your bike so that your toes just touch at the lower point in the pedaling cycle; this will ensure that your calf muscles relax and contract as you work. Swimming is also helpful, but it's not as effective as walking for pumping blood through the lower legs.

Walking, because it demands contraction of the calf muscle with each step, is the single most effective treatment I know of for reducing pain and minimizing discomfort caused by peripheral vascular disease. And walking offers an added benefit. There are latent and unused vessels in the body known as collaterals. Demand is the key to their utilization, and walking supplies it. As a result, small existing vessels may be widened to meet new demands, and in some cases latent or perhaps even new vessels may be opened and forced into service.

Whenever you walk, it is important that you have no other pain-producing problems in your lower limbs. The reason is basic: When you walk with pain you use more energy and burn more oxygen. So it is crucial that your shoes fit comfortably, and that you have no blisters or bunions, or bursitis of the heel.

If you suffer from peripheral vascular disease, you should, in consultation with your doctor, carefully consider the walking programs outlined in "Aerobic Activity." If you find that walking produces pain in your legs (as you make demands on your narrowed blood vessels), think of such discomfort as a sign that you are making progress. I remember one patient complaining of pain for whom I worked out a slightly nonmedical but nonetheless effective solution: a shot of whiskey (to dilate the blood vessels) followed by walking!

A drug was recently developed that actually changes the configuration of the red blood corpuscles and makes it easier for them to slip through the narrow arteries into the capillaries and thereby bring oxygen into the capillaries and to the tissues. We don't know enough about it yet, so I would urge you to go on a walking program as outlined.

Sometimes it is difficult to determine what the actual walking distance should be for the individual patient. Here is where a treadmill comes in handy. If you are uncertain about your walking tolerance, as you may well be, you should look for a rehabilitation department that conducts programs in peripheral vascular disease. They will determine, on a treadmill, exactly what your walking tolerance is and what incline you can handle. They will also make sure that you have no orthopedic condition which could increase the oxygen expenditure while you walk—a condition such as painful knees, heel spurs, pain in the front of your foot, low back pain, or very tight hips.

Walking is very important for peripheral vascular disease. If you have a musculoskeletal condition that prevents you from walking, there are many ways to overcome this condition. You may have to walk with a cane or some other device, but you should definitely walk! Peripheral vascular disease is something that we all face to some degree, but it is one of the few degenerative diseases in which the most effective treatment involves putting your best foot forward.

PHYSIATRICS

One advantage of being a physiatrist is that you can always get a conversation going merely by mentioning the word. "Physiatry" is a Greek term for the application of physical measures, and since most people are not familiar with it they start asking questions. Often I am mistaken, even at medical conferences and seminars, for the *psych*iatrist-in-chief of The New York Hospital–Cornell Medical Center. Such people must be puzzled as to why the psychiatrist-in-chief would be talking about injured shoulders and painful knees! At any rate, there are only 2,000 board-certified physiatrists in this country, specializing in the practice of physiatry or physiatrics. Its full name is really physical medicine and rehabilitation—"physical medicine" for the techniques we emphasize, which are *not* pharmacological or surgical, and "rehabilitation" for the process of recovery. Sometimes people refer to us as physical medicine doctors, other times as rehabilitation medicine doctors.

Heat, cold, water, electricity, exercise, prosthetics and orthotics, and a detailed functional analysis—these are the tools of physiatry. The usefulness of some of these techniques in treating human injury and illness was established hundreds of years ago, others more recently, but the underlying principle for all of them is the same: The human body is a *physical* system of remarkable versatility, and using physical means to help it heal itself is often the best and most effective kind of medicine.

Modern medical research has scored triumph after triumph, often with the aid of new medications, surgical breakthroughs, and space-age technologies, in the conquest of infection and other deadly forms of disease. Yet the body's bones and muscles, the levers and engines that rig and power the human machine and make up more than 50 percent of its mass, have been among the least studied of health care targets. Only a small fraction of the hours consumed by American medical education is devoted to nonsurgical approaches to the musculoskeletal system, and the concept of rehabilitation.

There are several reasons for this. Surgery and the use of medication have dominated health care in this country for many decades. Musculoskeletal problems, problems that are not usually dramatic or life threatening, do not always benefit from such approaches. In addition, soft-tissue ailments are difficult to diagnose, despite all the remarkable devices in the modern diagnostician's armory. And once a diagnosis is made, treatment may take weeks to months, progress is usually gradual, and quick, dramatic results are rare.

The irony is that problems involving physical disabilities are extremely common. According to the United States Bureau of the Census, more than 25 million Americans between the ages of eighteen and sixty-four now have a work disability, and another 10 million outside this age range also suffer from disabilities. Millions more, though not legally disabled, suffer from back, shoulder, knee, and elbow problems. It was recently reported that back pain is the second most common cause for hospitalization in the United States, next to childbirth. Other studies have determined that musculoskeletal ailments account for a major portion of all visits to doctors' offices, with some estimates ranging as high as 50 percent. Compounding the problem is the fact that as the American life span increases, the number of older people with physical ailments or disabilities will also rise so that the problem will become even more widespread. The forecast: Three out of four of us will suffer from a disabling physical condition at some point in our lives. Among people who are sixty-five years of age or older, a high percentage already require medication for various illnesses. Any healing approach such as ours, that reduces the need for additional medication, has to be advantageous.

At major medical centers, physiatry and its practitioners deal with major and often irreversible problems—paralysis, stroke, spinal cord damage, amputations, severe burns—and with nervous system disorders such as Parkinson's disease and multiple sclerosis, and with post-operative care following orthopedic or neurosurgical intervention. In private practice, physiatrists are more likely to treat soft-tissue ailments, such as low back muscular pain, and injuries related to sports and fitness and aftereffects of motor vehicle accidents, and work-related injuries. In both settings, however, the physiatrist brings to his patients a special awareness of the problems of joints, soft tissues, and pain, and loss of function. It is his job to make the patient as independent and active as possible, whether the disability is mild or severe. He requires a great deal of patience in handling such disorders. The physiatrist is not a surgeon, and unless absolutely necessary he relies less on medication than do other specialists, and more on exercise programs and other physical modalities of treatment. Progress may not always be rapid or dramatic, but physiatry works if the patient works with it.

In addition, physiatrists are trained to be experts in the use of electrodiagnostic studies, techniques designed to pinpoint the degree of damage in injured nerves and the extent to which muscles may suffer as a result. The functional capacity of nerves in the hands and face, the arms and legs, and between the ribs can be measured by these techniques, as can the effect of nerve damage on the muscles involved. With nerve damage there is relatively little that we can do to *promote* regeneration, but many nerves do come back, and with exercise we make sure that they have healthy muscle fibers to go to when they recover.

For some patients, especially those who have drifted from doctor to doctor in an attempt to ease their low back miseries or aching joints, physical medicine can be a revelation. In order to examine and diagnose a patient with a musculoskeletal problem, a physiatrist has to observe, touch (palpate), and move the body very carefully and thoroughly. He has to use the sensitivity of his fingertips the way a cardiologist uses his finely tuned ears to listen to heart sounds through a stethoscope. And once he has arrived at a diagnosis, he has to know how to prescribe an effective treatment program, drawing on the special techniques that are unique to his field.

Many people think that because ours is a very treatment-oriented specialty, and because many of our patients are referred to us by other physicians who have already

evaluated them, we don't need to establish a diagnosis. This is not true.

I recall a difficult case involving a young girl who was suffering from pain in her hip. Several physicians had seen her but could not agree on a diagnosis. The patient had been treated for rheumatoid arthritis, and a tissue sample had been taken to test for possible malignancy, but neither diagnosis could be substantiated. Her signs and symptoms—pain, weight loss, and pale color—continued. She consistently complained that she could feel something deep within her hip. The sedimentation rate of her red blood cells was elevated, suggesting an underlying though still unspecified disease process. Her X-rays, however, showed no abnormalities. I examined her on a number of occasions and found nothing. Then one day, after about a week, I noticed that her painful hip bulged slightly more than her other hip. Though the difference was just barely discernible, this was the clue that helped unravel the mystery. The girl had a benign cyst deep in the flesh of her hip, a pocket of infection that did not show up on X-rays and could only be detected by careful, daily observation.

One of our residents was in charge of another baffling case, even more difficult to diagnose than the hip cyst. A patient came to our department, a man who appeared to be in his late fifties or early sixties. He had a hoarse voice, he couldn't eat solid food, and he felt weak and listless. The patient had been tested with every device at New York Hospital, from CAT scan to bone scan, without any positive results. Our resident examined the patient, found nothing, and asked me what to do. I told her to sit the patient down, watch everything he did, and examine him until she found something. The resident was persistent and finally discovered, she thought, one muscle, the trapezius, that was weaker than the corresponding muscle on the other side of the man's body. She then performed an electrodiagnostic study and found a slight abnormality in the muscle, suggesting that something was irritating the nerve fibers supplying the muscles there. She had felt nothing over the area, but was convinced that something had to be pressing on a nerve. She began digging through anatomy books searching for possible answers. She gradually eliminated everything she could and wound up with the very tentative conclusion that a lymph node might be responsible for the patient's symptoms. After extensive discussion with a neurosurgeon, an exploratory operation was performed. During the procedure the surgeon removed an enlarged lymph node that indeed had been pressing on the nerve that controls the swallowing of food. If the node hadn't been located and cut out, the man's physical condition would have continued to deteriorate.

The point I want to make is not that physiatrists are capable of making diagnoses that other doctors don't make, but that physiatry examines the human body with extreme thoroughness and from every functional viewpoint because it has to. Even modern testing procedures are often inadequate in defining and detecting soft-tissue problems. Once a diagnosis is made, the physiatrist has at his disposal the physical agents and the techniques to help the body heal itself optimally with a minimum of functional deficit.

Which brings up another unique feature of a physiatrist's practice: the team of physical and occupational therapists with whom he works. The physiatrist is, in essence, besides being a physician, a team leader, drawing on all his medical knowledge and specialty training to develop and monitor the best possible treatment program for each patient. And while his medical education may have taken longer and been much more arduous and comprehensive than that of his therapists, the differences in their educational backgrounds become negligible when they are working together to help a patient. In fact, I rely very heavily on the information my therapists give me. There have even been times when they have helped me make a correct diagnosis. I can think of one recent case where a patient was being treated for some muscle spasms in the back, using our usual techniques. The physical therapist working with the patient was a conscientious and thorough observer who carefully examined each patient to monitor progress, but one day, after working with this particular patient for a few weeks, she came to me and reported that he seemed to have developed some difficulty walking, and that he also complained of some disturbances in his eyesight. She was concerned that he might have multiple sclerosis. She was right.

What exactly do physical therapists do? They receive their certification in one of two ways. Either they go to school after college for two or three years of intensive physical therapy courses, or they major in physical therapy at college—they must have a B.A. or B.S degree. They have expertise in teaching therapeutic exercise to patients, in handling machines that apply therapeutic agents, and knowledge in training patients how to use prosthetics and orthotics. They have a sound basis in anatomical and biomechanical principles, and they have to be skilled in dealing with people and sensitive to their personality traits and social circumstances.

In many centers, physical therapists participate in cardiac rehabilitation programs. Their special training in biomechanics and energy expenditure qualifies them to do this. Others may specialize in "chest physical therapy" to treat patients with breathing problems resulting from lung disease or post-operative compromise of lung function. They know how to position the patient properly, how to help train their respiratory muscles, how to free airways, and how to increase their tolerance to activity and exercise. Some of the therapists work exclusively with burn patients, helping to guide them through the most devastating period of their recovery, trying to prevent painful contractures, gradually helping them to increase their activities until they are ready to go home.

Another important member of the team is the occupational therapist, whose educational background is similar to that of the physical therapist. Unfortunately, the term "occupational therapist" is a misnomer. Occupational therapists do not give you *vocational* guidance or training. Rather, they are experts at making you as independent and functional in the real world as possible, in spite of your disability. For instance, if you have a stroke, an occupational therapist will work with you on balance and coordination and seemingly simple tasks like transferring you from the bed to the chair. He or she will teach you how to compensate for your disability with

special techniques or gadgets that can help you with everything from getting dressed to cooking or eating with a knife and fork. Occupational therapists have special expertise in working with hands and arms. If you have had your dominant arm amputated because of cancer, they will teach you how to do everything with the other hand. If one hand is weak, they can make "dynamic" splints for you from plastic materials or plaster casts so you can maximize the functions you still have. If you have lost feeling in your fingers and can't button your shirt, they will show you some tricks so you can do it yourself and not have to depend on anyone else. They also teach you special techniques to overcome swallowing difficulties, and are instrumental in the treatment of facial and upper-extremity burns.

Our Department of Rehabilitation Medicine also has a number of rehabilitation aides who are trained on the job to assist physical and occupational therapists with some of their more routine tasks. Their role is as important to the smooth operation of the team as that of all the other members.

Finally, patients who are hospitalized on a rehabilitation service, especially those with severe impairments who have to spend a long time in a rehabilitation center, are helped immeasurably by rehabilitation nurses, who have received special training in dealing with such patients.

Overnight miracles don't occur often in physiatry, but offering a good chance for maximum recovery through effective use of the resources that you, as the patient, possess are what makes this branch of medicine unique. You may be suffering from a painful tennis elbow or a pulled hamstring muscle, or you may have suffered the devastating consequences of a stroke or spinal cord injury. Whatever your ailment, it is important to remember that physical medicine and rehabilitation, working in tandem with more conventional medical treatments, operates to help you help yourself.

PLANTARIS TENDON RUPTURE

This is not a common injury, but it can occur—especially if you are active on the tennis court, or as a runner or jogger—and misdiagnosis often compounds the difficulty of obtaining proper treatment and adequate healing.

The plantaris muscle and its tendon run down through the lower leg behind the gastrocnemius (calf) muscle and is largely concerned with balancing the ankle as you move. When the tendon frays (it hardly ever ruptures completely), usually because you haven't warmed up properly or have overextended it, you will feel it go, most likely as a kind of pop or snap. Afterward, you may experience intense pain in the calf because of bleeding and formation of a hematoma (blood clot) at the site. The difficulty at this point is not determining whether or not you have suffered an injury—you know you have—but in determining exactly what that injury is.

One problem with diagnosis is that the plantaris tendon lies near the core of your lower leg, and this makes it hard to isolate and palpate the injured tissue. (Victims of the injury, because of the pain in the lower leg, sometimes think they have ripped their Achilles tendon, or have a severe case of shin splints.) If you were to come to my office with your painful leg, the first thing I'd do would be to listen to your story. Then, in what is known as the Thompson test, I'd ask you to lie on your stomach and raise your injured limb at the knee. I would gently squeeze your calf. If the sole of your foot were to move toward your back as I squeezed, I could be sure that your Achilles tendon was intact. If it were ruptured, you would not be able to move your foot. Assuming it is intact, I would next examine your leg, paying special attention to the area just below your calf muscle. This is where the plantaris muscle and its tendon join, and if I were to locate a painful knot at this point, I'd be reasonably sure that the plantaris muscle-tendon junction had been torn. In some such cases the calf muscle will be thrown into spasm, even though the muscle will not in fact be injured.

If the exam confirmed the diagnosis of plantaris tendon rupture, and if you were active on the tennis court and wanted to play again with the same level of balance, I would put you on crutches for one or two weeks, then on a cane for another week (and possibly on a heel lift for two to three weeks), until the frayed fibers had fully grown together with fibrous tissue. I would next start you on a program of exercises to loosen the calf muscle, because healing normally shortens muscle fibers. And, finally, I would put you on a rehabilitation program designed to strengthen both your plantaris and gastrocnemius muscles, along with any others that might have atrophied during inactivity. In another three or four weeks your plantaris tendon would be sound, and the muscle it serves would be as strong as before, perhaps even stronger.

I especially recommend such a careful and comprehensive approach for anyone forty years of age or older. Without such measures there is a higher likelihood that you will feel pain and stiffness in your lower leg for the rest of your life.

The Achilles tendon exercise program described earlier can also be used to stretch and strengthen your plantaris tendon, and should be done twice a day. Remember, stretching is important because the fibers in your tendon will have shortened as they healed. Be careful not to overstretch; this can rerupture fibers, especially in the early stages of the healing process. Be sure to breathe regularly while doing the exercises, and to relax completely between repetitions.

PLASTIC SURGERY AND FACIAL EXERCISES

Beauty may be only skin deep, but that doesn't make it any less important to many of us. For this reason, and because I believe strongly in personal improvement, I have few reservations about the cosmetic aspects of plastic surgery. If I did I would be hypocritical, for the desire to "look good" is often a doctor's best friend in motivating patients.

However, I do make it clear to patients who seek my advice that plastic surgery doesn't produce miracles. It will not make up for years of smoking, drinking, and unhealthy living. So you must be very realistic about what the results will be. Often in plastic surgery, human expectations are greater than the best results that can be

achieved by the most skilled hands. One should also realize that some cosmetic operations require a general anesthetic, and thus constitute major surgery with its attendant risks.

Having said this, I'll tell you about facial exercises as a possible supplement to the plastic surgeon's skill. The facts are brief. There are only two exercises for the face that are beneficial. Let me explain why.

Millions of muscle fibers arranged in groups and bundles provide the power that moves the body. These fibers are normally activated by the command of a nerve branch or a motor nerve. When orders come down to them from the brain through the spinal cord to perform a particular function, the appropriate nerve signals contraction, and fibers tighten. As a result, you may move your arm, kick a ball, or make a dash for the train. There are plenty of fibers ready to contract when necessary, and sufficient time for fibers that have contracted to remove waste products and recharge. But the ratio of nerve commanders to muscle-fiber soldiers varies from site to site. In the calf, for example, each motor nerve has about 1,200 fibers under its control; in the quadriceps the ratio may be one nerve to 400 to 600 muscle fibers. In the face, however, the ratio is down to one nerve to four to eight muscle fibers. This is the lowest in the body, and as a result, fatigue and exhaustion appear quickly in the face, and the facial muscles, if not used, are readily vulnerable to wasting away.

Because there are so few fibers in the face, it is also difficult to isolate muscle groups that can be strengthened by exercise. In fact, it can only be done in two areas. The exercises described below are designed to improve muscle tone in these areas.

These exercises are useful for both men and women, and should be done regularly, twice a day, in order to be of benefit. You can integrate the exercises into your morning and evening routines to help ensure your actually doing them. Do no more than 8 to 10 repetitions in each session. More repetitions will only tire out your facial muscles.

EXERCISE 1

This exercise will strengthen your cheek muscles and help prevent sagging in the lower part of your face. The exercise is

EXERCISE 1

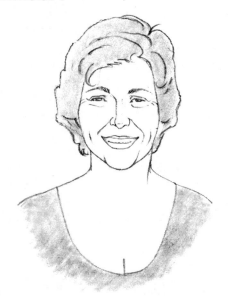

simple and common: a smile, but an exaggerated one that you hold for 5 seconds (count to 6), then relax for 2 seconds (count to 3). Do 8 to 10 repetitions morning and night, and be sure to perform the exercises daily.

EXERCISE 2

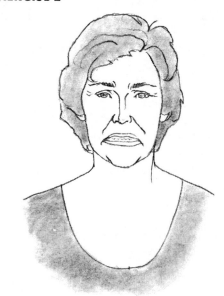

EXERCISE 2

This exercise is designed to strengthen your mentalis, or chin muscle. Instead of smiling as in the previous exercise, push your chin down and grimace, perhaps using a mirror to make sure that the corners of your mouth point downward. Hold each contraction for 5 seconds (count to 6), then relax for 2 seconds (count to 3). Do 8 to 10 repetitions morning and night, and be sure to perform the exercises daily.

POSTURE

The human spine curves four times as it descends from the skull to the coccyx. Two of these curves are pointed in toward the chest and two out toward the back. For the most part, modest deviations in this serpentine arrangement, which helps support the weight of the body and provides resilience, are natural. Some changes may be sculpted by the demands of work or the work environment, others by athletics or the pursuit of fitness, still others by the absence of any regular exercise at all. But the spine adapts well, and it will tolerate a great deal before it responds with pain and discomfort.

Viewed from the side, the spine first curves inward beneath the skull in a natural arch called lordosis. Here seven cervical vertebrae support the head and allow the neck to move. Then the spine swings out, and twelve thoracic vertebrae, which are attached to the ribs, make up this relatively rigid central portion of the back. An exaggeration of the thoracic curve is known as kyphosis. The spine's second inward curve occurs in the low back, or lumbar area, and five vertebrae, the body's largest, support everything above it. This natural curve is also known as lordosis, and when it is exaggerated the condition is called hyperlordosis, or swayback. The final curve is the sacrum, below the lumbar area. This second outward curve consists of five smaller vertebrae, fused together without disks in between, and the coccyx (four or five more small vertebrae) to complete the arc.

What constitutes good posture? Experts disagree even today, and throughout history hypotheses and programs designed to enhance health and fitness by straightening and strengthening the spine have intrigued if not always benefited man in his quest for self-improvement. Educators have been relatively dogmatic about correct posture, citing a familiar variation of military positioning with the shoulders back, chin down, and chest out. Now, however, there is less emphasis on rigid posturing and more on being lined up and forming a balanced and supportive unit from the head down to the legs.

Three fundamental posture-related problems can affect the spine and its curves. The first concerns osteoporosis, and the effect that bone thinning can have on the spinal vertebrae. In some cases, the vertebrae collapse as their bony structure becomes more and more compromised. This can lead to rounding of the shoulders and a kyphosis of the thoracic spine known as "dowager's hump." (The section on osteoporosis includes advice on calcium intake as well as impact exercises, and offers a program that will help you strengthen your back and shoulders and improve your appearance.)

The second problem is excessive inward arching of the lower back, the previously mentioned hyperlordosis. Weak abdominal muscles as well as poor posture can contribute to this condition, in which the pelvis tips forward, the lumbar curve is exaggerated, and the muscles that girdle and support the back are put under unnatural stress. The result: painful muscle tightness and spasm, the most frequent cause of low back miseries.

If you think you have or are susceptible to this problem, there is an easy way to check. Stand against a wall with your shoulders, buttocks, and heels touching it, reach behind your back with one hand and see if the hand slides *snugly* into your lumbar curve. If it does, you probably do not suffer from too much lordosis. But if your hand slips easily into the space, and there is room to move around, then the arch may be deeper than necessary and might cause problems in the future. In that case, I suggest you consider the low back exercise program presented at the end of this section. It will firm up your abdominal muscles, which are crucial in maintaining a strong and balanced back, and will loosen your hip flexors, allowing your pelvis to tip back into normal alignment and reducing the arch in your lower back.

The third posture problem involves younger children who, as they grow, may demonstrate a number of posture deviations that would be problematic if found in adults. Most will correct with time and normal childhood athletic activities, but if a child of about eight or nine consistently demonstrates a pronounced forward tilt of the head and neck, then it may be worthwhile to seek professional guidance.

How much deviation is too much? Have your child stand in a relaxed position, undressed and sideways, close to a white (and washable) wall, and cast a light to create a shadow profile of his posture. With a pencil, lightly trace the upper portion of this silhouette, then draw a vertical line up from the rearmost portion of the back. If the back of the child's head is more than four inches in front of this vertical line, then I would suggest you urge your child to do the exercise program outlined below. If you don't see any improvement after two

to three months, it would be a good idea to take the child to a physiatrist or exercise-oriented orthopedic surgeon for some modification of the exercise program.

It is relatively easy to correct posture abnormalities in younger people, but there is one kind of problem relating to the alignment of the spine that if left untreated can lead to painful and recurrent neck and shoulder problems in adulthood. This type of postural anomaly is in the lateral direction, and is most common in the age group between ten and twelve. If you look at your child and notice that one hip protrudes more than the other, or that the rib cage is somewhat asymmetrical, or that one shoulder blade protrudes more than the other when the child bends over, or there is an S-shape to the spine when you look at it from the back, I would urge you to consult a physiatrist or an orthopedic surgeon. Your child may have a condition known as scoliosis (girls are more frequently affected than boys), and both physiatrist and orthopedic surgeons have a special interest in its treatment. (See Scoliosis, page 234.) Or you could consult physicians in larger medical centers that have special clinics for scoliosis patients.

The following exercise program is designed to improve posture. Do not expect results overnight. It takes time and hard work to improve posture. The exercises must be done twice a day, every day, in a disciplined way. Just doing a few exercises once in a while will have no benefit. Remember to breathe regularly while exercising, and to relax completely between repetitions.

EXERCISE 1

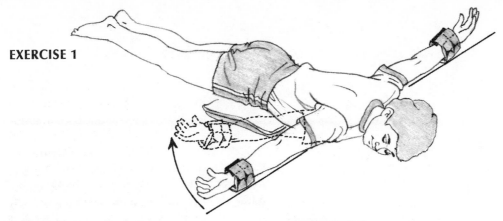

EXERCISE 1

This exercise is designed to build up the scapular adductors and the upper back extensors. Lie on your stomach with a pillow under your abdomen and a weight strapped to each wrist. Extend your arms out to the sides at shoulder height. Lift one hand at a time, hold for 5 seconds (count to 6), then lower and relax. Start off with a weight you can comfortably lift 8 times, and work up to 12 repetitions. Then add a pound and drop down to 8 repetitions, and gradually build up to 12 repetitions with 12 pounds.

EXERCISE 2

Here is another exercise to build up the scapular adductors and the upper back extensors. Lie on your stomach with a pillow under your abdomen and weights on your wrists. Extend your arms at a 45-degree angle to your body. Lift one hand at a time and hold for 5 seconds (count to 6), then lower and relax. Start off with a weight you can comfortably lift 8 times, and work up to 12 repetitions. Add a pound, drop down to 8 repetitions, and gradually build up to 12 repetitions with 12 pounds.

EXERCISE 2

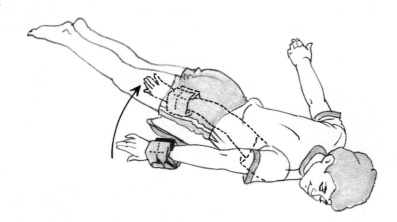

217

EXERCISE 3

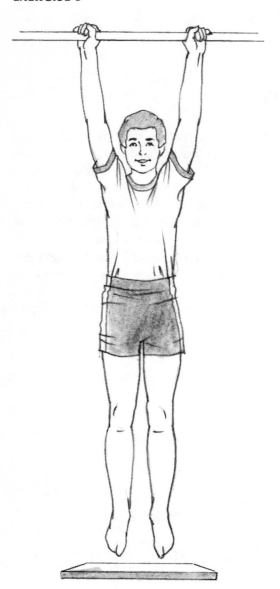

EXERCISE 3

Hanging from a bar is an excellent exercise for improving your posture, because it stretches the chest muscles. You should hang for 10 to 20 seconds. Try hanging for a few seconds at first, then resting, and then hanging again. Gradually build up the length of your "hang time" to one minute.

EXERCISE 4

This exercise requires pulleys. Most gyms and health clubs have them, or you can purchase a set from a sporting goods store. The following illustrations show the various pulley positions appropriate for different exercises. Stand with your back to the pulleys, grab the handles behind you with the palms facing away from the apparatus, then pull the weights forward. Start off doing 15 repetitions of 4 pounds. When this becomes easy, add 2 pounds. Your goal is eventually to do 15 repetitions of 10 pounds. If you don't have access to pulleys, you can do the same exercise with free weights, reducing the poundage by half. Be sure to relax for a second after each repetition, otherwise you will tighten your muscles.

EXERCISE 5

Stand with your back to the pulleys, grab a handle with each hand, then pull your arms down and toward the floor. Relax and repeat as in the previous exercise.

EXERCISE 4

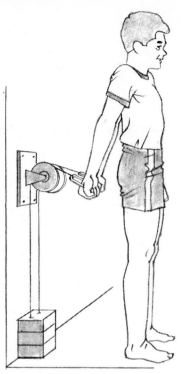 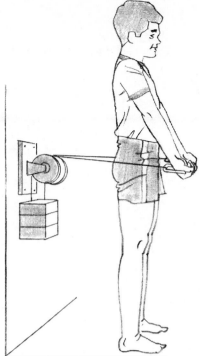

EXERCISE 5

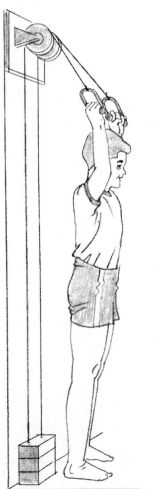 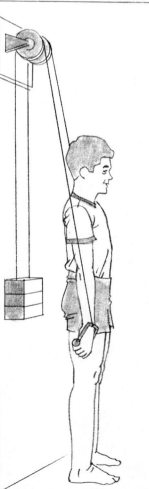

EXERCISE 6

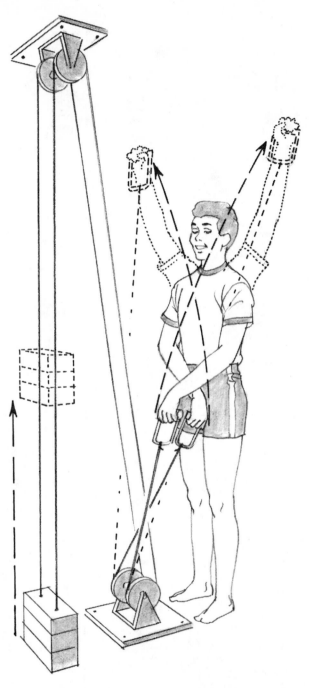

EXERCSISE 6

Also done with pulleys, this exercise strengthens your upper back extensors and scapular adductors. Stand facing the pulleys. Holding the pulley handles, cross your hands at groin level and pull your arms up and out so that they come up over your head and spread out to the sides. Relax and repeat as in the preceding exercises.

EXERCISE 7

This exercise is designed to stengthen your upper back extensors, and make you more posture conscious. Stand with your back touching a wall, then use the muscles in your shoulders to brace your shoulders and head back against the wall. This should make your shoulder blades move closer together. Hold for 5 seconds (count to 6), then relax for 2 seconds (count to 3). Do 12 repetitions.

EXERCISE 7

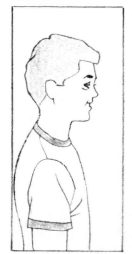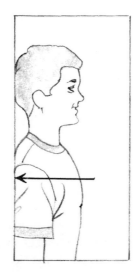

EXERCISE 8

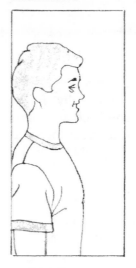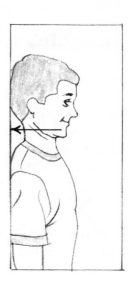

EXERCISE 8

This exercise stretches the back neck muscles and strengthens those in front. Stand near a wall or sit in a straight-backed chair with your feet flat on the floor and your arms relaxed at your sides. Your head should be level. Slowly tuck your chin into your neck as far as you can. Hold this position for 5 seconds (count to 6), then relax for 2 seconds (count to 3). Do not bring your chin down toward your chest, or flex your head forward. You should feel a pull in the back of your neck. Repeat this exercise 5 times.

PRONATION AND SUPINATION

These often confused terms may be vaguely familiar to you, especially if you are a runner or jogger. This is because they refer to the manner in which your foot and arch hit the ground and distribute weight when you run (or walk, for that matter), whether casually or at competitive-distance speeds.

During regular human locomotion (anything up to sprinting), the heel of the foot strikes the ground first, then the body's weight shifts to the outside of the foot (supination), and finally the arch flattens and weight is spread to the inside of the foot (pronation).

Though all three steps—heel touch, supination, and pronation—are normal parts of the gait cycle, exaggeration of any of them can cause problems, though not necessarily in the foot. Runners with flat or flattening arches, for example, will have an early and exaggerated heel strike, leading to bruising and tendon trouble in the area. Such a condition can also transmit impact up the leg and cause pain on the inside of the knee. Excessive supination, or pronation, can also lead to painful knee problems.

One way to check the impact pattern of your feet is to examine your running shoes. If they show wear on the outside edge of the sole, you tend to supinate; if the wear is on the inside, you tend to pronate. Another simple exam can be conducted at the beach. If you step carefully in firm sand, your print will show little sign of an arch,

in the case of pronation; if you supinate, only the outer part of your foot will be imprinted.

The important thing to remember is that we all pronate and supinate to some degree, and that many athletes with either of these abnormalities still perform without difficulty. Problems that do result from imperfect weight distribution can usually be alleviated by custom-made inserts for your shoes and your running and tennis footgear. Specialists in the field of orthotics create such corrective devices, and most are extremely effective in redistributing body weight and reducing pain and injury.

RADIATION AND PHYSICAL ACTIVITY

Enormous advances have been made in the technique of therapeutic radiation and in improving its efficiency. Many malignant or potentially malignant conditions are now treated with radiation alone or in connection with surgery or chemotherapy, and the side effects that often used to complicate treatment, such as radiation burns, can now be prevented or at least forestalled.

If you have to undergo radiation treatment, you may wonder what adjustments, if any, you should make with regard to physical activity. Having treated many patients while they were receiving radiation, and having seen many musculoskeletal complications from radiation, which I believe could have been prevented, I would advise the following: If you receive radiation to a certain part of your body, you should by all means keep this part active, if not in the course of your daily activities, then as part of a formal exercise program. For example, in the case of radiation to the shoulder or to the axilla, for carcinoma of the breast, I strongly advise exercising the shoulder every day. Some of these exercises may turn out to be superfluous, but they will take only a few minutes a day and will certainly help prevent a frozen shoulder. After radiation, some of the connective tissue can tighten up and start to restrict one's range of motion, so it is all the more important to keep the radiated body part active.

One complication of radiation is osteoporosis, or an eventual weakening of the bone structure. Again, the best preventive measure is to stay very active so that bone metabolism will be stimulated. My experience is that the more active you are, the less likely you are to suffer from the ill-effects of osteoporosis. Of course, one cannot entirely prevent the osteoporotic changes that come about with radiation. For instance, if you receive radiation to the lungs and it includes the vertebrae of the spine, you may develop osteoporosis of the vertebrae, which could lead to compression fractures.

Still, whatever your case, I would recommend very strongly that you stay active, that you keep on playing golf or tennis or swimming, and walking. You can also undertake other formal exercises, whatever you can tolerate. I would only avoid jumping, weightlifting, prying open windows, or other activities that involve a sudden stress or prolonged and increasing stress. Just don't be inactive—it will only encourage osteoporotic changes. If you have any questions, speak to a physiatrist who can advise you on your activities and exercises.

A particularly vulnerable area during and after radiation treatment is the hip area. Radiation-induced osteoporotic changes in the neck of the thigh bone, near the pelvis, increase the risk of hip fracture, so one should stay active in a way that regularly stresses the bone to help it deposit minerals, mostly calcium. It may also help to take a calcium supplement (except in cases where there is also disease of the kidneys).

In the event someone experiences pain in the hip after radiation treatments, they should consult a physiatrist or an orthopedic surgeon who will make a decision about further care. It is entirely possible that prophylactic or preventive internal fixation ("nailing") of the hip will have to be employed. I have not seen any serious complication with this procedure, as long as the necessary precautions were taken.

Not everyone who receives radiation eventually suffers from osteoporosis, and even those who do, do not necessarily suffer any ill effects as long as they care for the problem properly by staying active and avoiding extreme stress.

RHEUMATOID ARTHRITIS

There is an enormous difference between osteoarthritis and rheumatoid arthritis. Osteoarthritis is an age-related and extremely common affliction (most of us have some, but don't always know it) that attacks the joints, roughening them, inhibiting motion, and causing stiffness and pain. Rheumatoid arthritis (RA) is a "systemic" disease involving many parts and systems of the body *besides* the joints. It is by far the more serious ailment, for it means that you won't simply have a sore knee or stiff hip but that your whole body will be under attack. When I see osteoarthritis patients, they often turn out to be vigorous and strong and tell me, "I'm in good health and nothing bothers me but my hip, which hurts all the time." Rheumatoid patients, on the other hand, tend to come in to my office with more serious problems.

More than 5 million adult Americans are now afflicted with rheumatoid arthritis, and though researchers have grappled with the problem for decades, there is no cure and no clear understanding of its causes. There is a leading "player," however, and that is the immune system. Normally, this system protects the body against outside invaders; however, in certain instances it turns and attacks its own tissues. Rheumatoid arthritis, like osteoarthritis, involves destruction of the cartilage, but a rheumatoid problem actually starts in the synovial, or fluid-producing, membrane that lines and lubricates the joints. This destructive process can affect adjacent bones and ligaments as well as tendons and muscles, creating a great deal of instability and sometimes causing severe deformity of the joints. Joints in the hands, knees, and feet are most often involved, though rheumatoid arthritis may also affect the blood vessels, the lungs, the spleen, the eyes, even the heart. Sufferers may go through long periods of remission and then experience a severe attack lasting several weeks. Such attacks seem to appear most frequently when the immune system is functioning poorly because of a cold or fatigue or emotional stress.

Not every one diagnosed as having rheumatoid arthritis faces severe disability, however, and many recover completely after one or more attacks. Others may suffer from several bouts of inflammation, usually widely spaced and of varying degrees of intensity. Still, less than 10 percent of those with the disease wind up being severely disabled by it. And even this is a negotiable statistic, for new research programs are being launched constantly, new drugs are being tested, and existing medications—ranging from heavy doses of aspirin to the use of cortisone and even gold—can be highly effective. I would strongly recommend that you keep in touch with an experienced rheumatologist (a specialist in joint disease) who will adjust your medication according to your needs.

An important consideration if you have been diagnosed as having rheumatoid arthritis is to realize that besides taking medication there are many things you *can* do, and if you work to build up your body after a rheumatoid arthritis attack, you'll have a much greater capacity to withstand the ravages of the next one. The human body can withstand a great deal of skeletal abnormality if its muscular system is well-tuned and strong. You may not be able to do much when suffering a flare-up, but if you work with an experienced physiatrist between attacks you can accomplish a great deal.

Let me explain how and why in greater detail. If your muscles are not well trained and you go to do something, you bring into play many more fibers than you actually need in order to perform the task. This sort of muscular overkill puts pressure on your tendons, the cartilage in your joints, and the joints themselves, which may already be tender. In general, you make an already bad situation worse. But if your muscles are trained, you may need the contraction of just one or two muscle groups to perform the same task. This makes it easier for you to do normal things, and it lightens any load where it most needs to be lightened: on your joints. Along with a carefully structured exercise program, general health maintenance measures are very important.

I am not going to provide any exercise instructions here because each rheumatoid arthritis patient must have a highly individualized program adjusted according to the extent and severity of the disease. Because the muscles themselves are affected by the disease process, they will respond differently than they would in the case of an osteoarthritic patient. Any rheumatoid exercises will therefore be much more gentle, and it will take longer for the muscles to show signs of improvement.

I should add that for acute attacks, special splints can be fabricated by occupational therapists to protect the inflamed joints. If the joints become so deformed that you actually lose the use of your hands, the therapists can evaluate you for all sorts of adaptive equipment to compensate.

So, much can be done to temper the ill effects of this insidious disease, though it does require expert guidance, provided either by a physiatrist experienced in the treatment of RA patients or by an exercise-oriented rheumatologist.

ROTATOR CUFF TEAR

This has become an impressive, even fearful, term in these days of sports-medicine awareness, but unless you make your living pitching for a professional baseball team you really don't have much to worry about. The words *rotator* and *cuff* are used to designate the function and structure of three small shoulder muscles: the supraspinatus, the infraspinatus, and the teres minor. Together they cap your shoulder and bind your ball-and-socket arm joint in place while permitting rotation. And, yes, you can tear or, in most instances, partially tear one of these muscles or its muscle-tendon connection, even if you don't make a living playing baseball. But the truth is that in 95 percent of such cases, if you work to maintain the range of motion in your shoulder and the strength of your muscles, the damage will heal on its own, without surgery.

A violent, vigorous reaching motion—jerking a heavy suitcase off a luggage carousel, for example—is most likely to cause a tear. But you can rip your rotator cuff under a variety of conditions and unexpected moments. I once had a patient who injured his shoulder while he was in the hospital, sitting in bed! He had just undergone surgery for another problem and, being a bit impatient, he tried to push his IV pole out of the way. Unfortunately, the pole was anchored to the floor, and when it wouldn't move he gave it a hard yank. The pole remained rooted, but the muscles in his rotator cuff didn't! He told me later, "I knew I tore something as soon as it happened."

You, too, will probably know if you suffer this kind of injury. You may not feel much pain, but you are likely to hear or feel something pop. This information would be important for me to have as your physician, because it is not always easy to make the correct diagnosis when it comes to shoulder pain. Your shoulder, especially as you grow older, may suffer from any number of problems, all of which can cause pain in the joint connection or capsule. You may, for example, have overused your arm or irritated the bursae, the small sacs that help lubricate the rotator cuff muscles where they attach to bone.

The first thing that I would do in such a case is make sure that you haven't suffered nerve damage, and that the nerves in your neck and shoulder are all functioning normally. Then, especially if you have told me that a sudden jerking motion launched the problem, I would examine the range of motion in your shoulder. I might ask you to place your hands on your chest and, keeping your shoulders down, raise your elbows as high as you could. If one of your shoulders were weak or stiff, then the crest of that shoulder would bulge close to your neck as you tried to compensate for the weakness of your rotator cuff muscles. If I asked you to hold your arms out—parallel to the floor with elbows bent at a 90-degree angle and palms down—and then told you to press down on my hands, I might detect weakness in one arm. This could indicate a

loss of strength from rotator cuff damage. If I then asked you to raise your arm straight out to the side and up, then slowly lower it, and your arm gave way quickly during the last 10 or 15 degrees, being too weak to control this motion, you would likely have torn your rotator cuff muscles.

If there were reason to believe that you had suffered a complete tear, I would recommend having an arthrogram. This is an invasive procedure that involves injecting an opaque dye into the shoulder joint prior to X-raying the area in order to see the surrounding structures more clearly. If surgery is not absolutely indicated—and in most rotator cuff injuries it is not—I consider an arthrogram superfluous. A therapeutic exercise program is based on physical findings, and I know of no case where an arthrogram was helpful in designing such a program. In actual practice, my feelings would change only if you were a professional athlete whose livelihood depended on your shoulder functioning properly. A more aggressive approach with surgical intervention would, in that case, save you some valuable time.

Once the diagnosis had been established and it was determined that you were not a candidate for surgery, I would suggest that you keep moving the shoulder, using the exercises that follow, and wait for the tear to heal itself. If the damage were extensive, then I might suggest putting your arm in a sling for a few days. In all, healing would probably take about six to eight weeks. That may seem a long time, but fast healing requires a good blood supply, and the supply to the rotator cuff muscles is poor.

The results of an exercise program for a rotator cuff tear can be just as good as those produced by surgery and you face fewer risks. Letting the body, aided by proper exercise, heal itself, is often the best medicine. The problem, in this age of abundant medication and impressive surgical opportunities, is knowing when an exercise program will do the job just as effectively.

If you think you have torn something in your shoulder, a physiatrist or an orthopedic surgeon is probably the best person to see, and if your primary physician refers you to a specialist for further management, a physiatrist is certainly worthwhile to guide you in an exercise program. An orthopedic surgeon could also do this, but if an arthrogram and surgery are recommended, I strongly suggest you consider a nonsurgical approach instead. You nearly always try a rehabilitation program first, and then, if it's not as effective as anticipated, try surgery.

The exercises that follow are designed to keep your rotator cuff muscles loose and to gradually strengthen them as they heal. By making your muscles both looser and stronger, you will be much less likely to suffer further big-league injuries.

EXERCISE 1

This exercise strengthens the external rotators and assumes you have injured the rotator cuff of your right shoulder. Lie on your left side, on a bed or couch, and support your head with your left hand. Holding a 1-pound weight in your right hand, place that hand at your waist with elbow bent. Raise and straighten the arm out to the side, behind your body and parallel to the floor. Hold for 5 seconds (count to 6), then return to original position and relax for 3 seconds (count to 4). Start off doing 8 repetitions and work up to 12. When you can do 12 repetitions comfortably, increase the weight by a pound, drop back to 8 repetitions, and work your way back up to 12 repetitions with 10 pounds.

EXERCISE 1

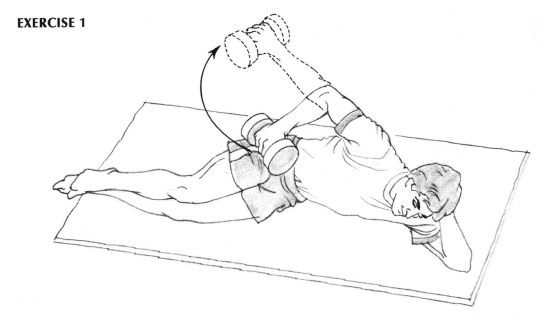

EXERCISE 2

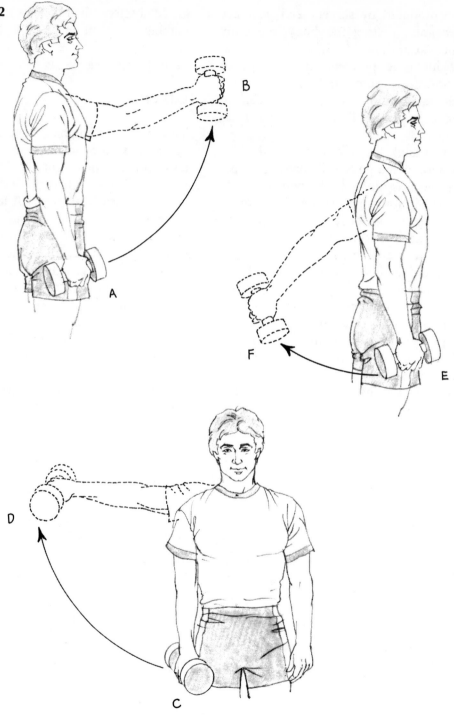

EXERCISE 2

It is also important to maintain strength in the deltoid muscle, which weakens quickly when you don't move your shoulder normally. This exercise works on all three components of the deltoid muscle—the anterior, middle, and posterior. Start with a 3-pound weight. Stand erect with your arm at your side, raise your straight arm up to shoulder level in front of your body (a–b). Work as in the previous exercise, holding each repetition for 5 seconds (count to 6), then lowering the arm and relaxing for 2 seconds (count to 3). This strengthens the anterior component. Next, from the same starting position, raise the arm out to the side as far as you can without straining—this strengthens the medial component (c–d). Finally, again from the same starting position, raise the arm behind you to strengthen the posterior component (e–f). Be careful not to force your arm too far backward. Start off with 8 repetitions in each direction and work up to 12. When you can easily perform 12 repetitions in each direction, add a pound and drop down to 8 repetitions. Increase the weight gradually until you can do all three phases of the exercise with 10 pounds for 12 repetitions. If the deltoid muscle proves weak or your shoulder becomes painful, rest the weight on a table and loosen your grip on it between repetitions.

EXERCISE 3

This exercise is to strengthen the supraspinatus and deltoid muscles, muscles that may not be injured in a rotator cuff tear,

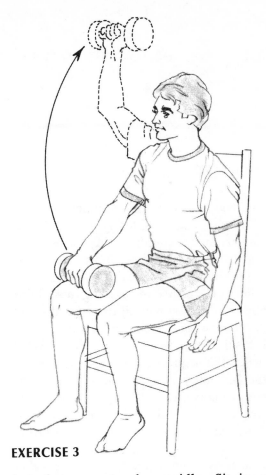

EXERCISE 3

but that can atrophy rapidly. Sit in a straight-backed chair with your feet flat on the floor and a 1- to 3-pound weight in hand resting palm down in your lap. Extend your arm out toward your knee, then raise it straight up until it is over your head. Start off doing 8 repetitions and work up to 12; hold each for 5 seconds (count to 6). When you can do 12 repetitions easily, add one pound, drop down to 8 repetitions, and work back up to 12 repetitions and a total of 12 pounds. Each repetition should take 5 seconds (count to 6), and you should relax for 2 seconds (count to 3) between repetitions. You can rest the weight on a table as in the preceding exercise.

229

RUNNER'S KNEE

The body has one very common problem of overuse, and considering the number of runners in this country today, it's surprising that it doesn't occur more frequently.

Let's look at the realities of running a mile. In the course of covering those 1,482 meters, your feet will hit the ground about 2,000 times, and each time a foot lands it bears the entire weight of your body. What makes this sequence even more amazing is the fact that your weight at impact will be considerably greater than your actual body weight. As a result of forward speed and downward velocity, the total will probably be between two and a half to three times your body weight. What this means is that if you weigh 150 pounds and run a mile, you will, by conservative estimate, land on each foot with an aggregate weight of more than 400 tons during that one mile. This is an awesome figure, of course, but the body is generally designed well enough to absorb and distribute such stress.

There are two different kinds of physical problems that can cause pain and discomfort in the knee after running—the pain is usually right around the kneecap, sometimes just to each side of it. The first problem involves the arch of the foot. If this intricate structure is lower than normal, or flat, and thus is relatively inflexible when the foot comes down, the result may be pain in the knee as impact is transmitted up the leg and into the joint. The same thing can happen with an arch that is high and inflexible, with pain occurring either in the knee or, in some cases, in the heel.

The second kind of physical problem that leads to knee pain in runners involves the alignment of the leg, knee, and foot. In some cases your leg may angle inward and your foot turn under slightly (or supinate). You can check for this condition by examining the wear pattern on the bottom of your running shoes. If the outer edge of the shoe is worn down, it's an indication that you tend to supinate when you run. This may not be a problem for the foot, but it can, in certain cases, deliver stress to your knee. It is also possible that you may pronate, which means that the wear and tear will be on the inside of your foot and shoe rather than the outside. This inside-out twisting can also deliver unusual stresses to the knee area—in the tendon that runs over the knee cap, for example, or in the pes anserinus tendons (so-called in Latin because when dissected they resemble a goose's foot), which lie on the inside of the knee and attach the hamstrings to the tibia, the large bone in the lower leg.

In instances of protracted swelling, inflammation, tendinitis, and nonspecific pain in the knee, my advice is to stop running for a few days and have the knee evaluated by a physiatrist or orthopedic surgeon. Medication can help temporarily, but the important thing is to get a thorough evaluation, one that will pinpoint and distinguish overuse difficulties from ligament or cartilage damage, and both from structural anomalies.

Aspirin and other anti-inflammatory medications can help with inflammation, but rest is just as important, and of even greater value is the manner in which you return to jogging or running. Whatever you do, don't resume at the level at which you stopped. My rule of thumb is: Double the time you have been out of action and use that period to work back up to your original level of activity. If you've been out one week, take two to get back; if you've been out two, take a month. And start your return by doing a quarter of what you were doing before you stopped.

If evaluation turns up ligament or cartilage damage in your knee, which is always possible, remember that surgical intervention, even when it involves modern arthroscopic techniques, should be considered as a last resort. Many of the new sports medicine procedures sound good and have received considerable publicity, but this does not mean that they are right for you (unless you are a competitive athlete) or that in the long run they will be more beneficial than conservative measures.

Arthroscopy is a great advantage over the old type of surgery—where the knee had to be opened up to a much greater extent—and the post-operative recovery time is much shorter. I recommend arthroscopy for cartilage injuries only if: (1) there is jamming of the joint line, and rest, ice, and keeping your weight off the knee do not help unlock it; and (2) the pain returns with resumption of activity after an apparently successful knee rehabilitation program—that is, with full range of motion and quadriceps strength restored.

Unless you fall into these categories, my advice is to rest your knee first, then work to build up the muscles, the quadriceps, and hamstrings that provide 30 percent of the joint's stability. Running uphill and climbing stairs are good ways to strengthen your hamstrings, but I would advise against downhill running. That puts much more stress on your knee and can lead to substantial injury. Stress fractures of the tibia and bones in the feet happen much more frequently from running downhill than uphill.

If knee surgery is necessary, try to build up your natural physical resources first. Remember that muscles have a memory, and if the muscles were well-trained and strong before the injury, your rehabilitation will proceed much more quickly. Athletic activities should not be resumed before quadriceps strength has been regained and is at least as strong on the injured leg as on the sound one. Once you become involved in running again, you should consider using a protective knee brace with enforcements on the inner and outer sides. This does not give true mechanical support, but it does distribute stresses on the knee more favorably.

Treatment for problems that involve structural anomalies most often leads to the specialty known as orthotics, the science that creates custom-made supports designed to realign the foot, ankle, and leg, if the problem involves pronation, supination, or low or high arches. The result is a more natural distribution of the stresses generated by running or other forms of vigorous activity that involve continual pounding. Such devices may be somewhat expensive, but in most cases they are well worth the cost. This is an instance, and an important one, in which man-made devices can help fine-tune the human machine and make it run more smoothly for a longer time.

RUNNING SHOES

As you get older, it is highly likely that one foot or both feet will acquire some slight abnormalities, and while this may not cause you any major problems, you might find that one foot fits into shoes less well than the other. (Most of us don't have completely equal feet anyway.) It is entirely possible that you need two different sizes, available from many shoe stores that have a big selection of sneakers.

What should you look for? The shoes should have a flexible sole for the ball of the foot. You should be able to bend the sole easily with your hand; otherwise, you will not have enough propelling action from your toes when you are running, particularly when running fast, which will put a lot of stress on the ball of your foot. The shoes should also have a rather snug cuff. There should be no sideways motion, and you should be able to wiggle your toes easily to allow for your feet enlarging slightly as you run (caused by the blood supply increasing about ten to fifteen times). Allow extra room in the shoe for the longest toe, usually the first or second toe.

If you should happen to get your shoes wet when you run, either on wet grass or in the rain, my advice is either to put in some shoe stretchers afterward or to fill the shoes with newspaper and let them air dry. Don't put them on a radiator or in a clothes dryer. Your shoes will become very stiff if you do this, and lose some of their configuration. Ill-fitting shoes can be the cause of all kinds of foot problems likely to interfere with your running schedule.

SCANNERS

A CAT (computerized axial tomography) or CTT (computerized transaxial tomography) scanner, is a very sophisticated device that creates remarkably sharp cross-sectional pictures of anatomical structures, in contrast to X-rays, which are two-dimensional and do not tell you much about soft-tissue structures. The system constructs such pictures by taking a series of X-rays from a variety of angles. This information is reassembled by the scanner's computer to produce accurate cross-sectional images. In the Department of Rehabilitation Medicine at The New York Hospital–Cornell Medical Center, we are likely to use CAT scans to confirm clinically based diagnoses of problems in the lumbar, or lower spinal, region, including disk abnormalities and spinal stenosis. Occasionally, we may scan the cervical or upper spine for the same type of problem, though with less success, the reason being that the neck carries less fatty tissue than the lumbar spine and the images are not as clearly defined.

In the days before the CAT scan, we used myelograms rather routinely to obtain the same kind of information. However, myelograms are an invasive technique that involves injecting a dye into the spinal canal and carries with it the risk of causing pain, discomfort, and temporary disability. A CAT scan allows physicians to look inside the body without doing anything invasive. Sometimes a dye is used with the CAT scan to help delineate delicate structures, but the dye in this case is injected into a vein and not the spinal canal.

The NMR (nuclear magnetic resonance) scanner is an even more sophisticated device that utilizes a large doughnut-shaped magnet. The magnet manipulates the nuclei of certain atoms in the patient's cells, and, along with radio waves, creates high-resolution pictures of various body systems, including nerves and muscles. Still in its developmental stages, the NMR scanner is already very useful in diagnosing neurological diseases such as multiple sclerosis and brain tumors. As far as the physiatrist and rehabilitation medicine are concerned, however, the CAT scan is still a more valuable tool. We have tried to use the NMR scan for documenting lumbar spinal disorders, but at its present stage of development it has not reached the diagnostic usefulness of the CAT scan. So far, the NMR belongs more in the sphere of the neurologist and neurosurgeon than the physiatrist.

There are also PET (positron emission tomography) scanners. These machines are capable of indicating how cells make use of the fuels they consume. A PET scanner can indicate oxygen intake, the accumulation of calcium, and other types of extremely delicate metabolic changes. In the future, when the machines become useful at the clinical level, this type of information may be of crucial importance in the diagnosis and treatment of a variety of injuries and illnesses, including those involving the brain's cells and tissues.

SCIATICA

The sciatic nerves, the body's largest, originate in the lower back and actually consist of two pairs of nerves—one for each leg. Each pair of nerves travels in one sheath through the buttocks and down the back of the thigh to the back of the knees. Here its two components divide and travel separately down into the calf and foot. Over the years, the term "sciatica" has come to refer to almost any kind of pain that involves the back and legs, when it should in fact be applied only to discomfort caused by irritation or pressure on the sciatic nerve or on the roots of its trunk.

The pain can be either sharp and extremely debilitating, or a dull ache, and it can involve one leg or both. Sciatic pain created by pressure on or irritation of the roots that form the nerve as they emerge from the vertebral column may originate in one of three ways.

First, the surfaces of the vertebrae may become roughened with age, and at certain times—especially in later life when the disks are thinner and the vertebrae come closer together—bony spurs may press on the sciatic nerve and cause radiating pain. This may occur in certain positions, such as leaning back while walking downhill, or sleeping on your stomach, which arches your back.

The second cause of pressure on sciatic nerve roots may involve the disks themselves, which normally cushion the vertebrae and function as soft-tissue shock absorbers. Occasionally, the tough outer covering of a disk will tear and bulge, and in some instances the soft inner filling will ooze out and actually press on the sciatic nerve. Pain caused by disk pressure is similar to that triggered by bony spurs.

A third cause of sciatic pain, and one that is often overlooked, is muscular in origin. Muscle spasms or trigger points in the vicinity of the nerve may be responsible for irritating the nerve anywhere along its course. This is most often true for the piriformis muscle, which lies deep within the buttock and may go into spasm and tighten to such a degree that it presses on the sciatic nerve and causes pain. A tip-off to this syndrome is the fact that there is usually no pain above the buttock muscles.

Certain malignancies may also trigger sciatic pain when they impinge on the nerve. As a result, a specific diagnosis is very important and not always easy to establish. I would recommend that you go to a physiatrist or to a neurologist with special experience in treating back problems. Once the possibility of a malignancy has been ruled out, a conservative or nonsurgical treatment can be initiated in most instances. Surgical intervention is used less frequently these days in treating sciatica, and there is little evidence that traction helps. In many cases, however, a specific exercise program can help reduce pressure on the nerves by strengthening weak muscles and loosening tight ones. This allows the pelvis to assume a more natural position, one that should improve nerve passage through the foramina. Trigger points, if present, can be released with injections and physical therapy.

Attacks of sciatica can be painful and disturbing, and if you experience one, I would advise you to immediately lie down on a firm mattress, with one or two pillows under your knees. Such positioning should help relieve the pain somewhat. Remember that though the pain may be very upsetting, nothing of a life-threatening nature is going to happen to you. If muscle spasms are involved, try ice and some gentle limbering exercises.

If osteoarthritic changes are the cause of irritation of the sciatic nerve, you can try some anti-inflammatory medication and some pain medication. As the acute stage subsides somewhat, you can also start with some gentle limbering exercises. It is important to keep in mind that most back pain episodes do not lead to surgery, and that a myelogram is not usually necessary unless surgery is being contemplated.

If, on careful physical examination, a trigger point (see Trigger Points, page 268) is detected in the area of the piriformis muscle, it should be injected and treated with the usual therapy of electrical stimulation, ice, and massage. The treatment of piriformis muscle tightness is not so easy— it can take longer to relax this particular muscle than many others in the lower back and hip region—but the results will be all the more gratifying once achieved.

SCOLIOSIS

Scoliosis is a sideward curvature and rotation of the lumbar or thoracic spine. The origin of this curvature is not known yet, but one theory holds that it is caused by muscular imbalances. Very often it is not the sideward curvature of the spine that is noticed first, but an inequality of the rib cage—that is, the rib cage sticks out on one side further than on the other, always on the side of the convexity. It usually occurs between age ten and twelve, and is much more prevalent in girls than in boys. (When adults have X-rays taken of their lumbar or thoracic spine for some painful condition, the X-ray report may mention a scoliotic curve. Such a report often raises concern, but it is most likely a coincidental finding and not contributory to the patient's complaints. Millions of people have "a little bit of scoliosis.")

How can one detect childhood scoliosis? Since teenagers are usually shy and don't want to get undressed in front of their parents, it is often discovered by the school nurse. One way of finding out is to ask your son or daughter to stand undressed and bend forward and then come up slowly. Notice whether the curvature of the spine is in the upper thoracic area or in the lumbar area, or in both. Often one can see an asymmetry of the back muscles, where one side is more developed than the other. Occasionally, both thoracic and lumbar curvatures are about equal and compensate each other; we then speak about a "compensated scoliosis," which means if a plumb line were taken from the head it would fall right into the midline of the sacrum—the bone at the base of your back.

Once you have discovered your child has scoliosis, what do you do about it? He or she should be seen by an orthopedic surgeon, or a physiatrist who deals in this area, and an X-ray should be taken. But then comes the most important part. Don't restrict your child. Most children with scoliosis can perform physical activities quite well, and only if there is an extreme curvature—over 40 or 50 degrees—can physical performance be impaired.

There are different views about the treatment of scoliosis. My experience is that the curvature cannot be changed with exercise, although developing very strong trunk, stomach, and shoulder muscles, and a high aerobic capacity will decrease the chances of later pain. There will be an increased stress on the muscles because of the curvature of the spine, and a well-trained body can withstand such stress much better. Nearly all sports can be performed to a high level by persons with scoliosis, particularly symmetrical sports such as swimming. I advise against pressing weights, though weight exercises in the supine position or with handweights are advisable. The goal has to be to strengthen the back extensor muscles, as well as the shoulder, stomach, and leg muscles.

Some physicians and therapists may recommend so-called rotational and derotational exercises for scoliosis patients, but I never saw anyone who derived any benefit from them.

The mistake of overprotection often occurs with scoliotic children. Girls are usually more concerned than boys about cosmetic appearances. The curve should be checked yearly with X-rays and preferably by the same physician who did the original examination. The reproductive organs ought to be protected carefully when taking X-rays. Once the growth period is over, between eighteen and twenty-one, I don't think yearly checks are indicated, although the patient should still be seen perhaps every other year by a scoliosis specialist.

Various treatments for scoliosis are available. One of the most favored for extreme cases is Harrington rod surgery, where the spine is actually straightened out with steel rods. Another treatment is the so-called scoliosis brace, also known as the Milwaukee brace. Other forms of braces are also available. They all have to be worn for years, and practically all day, and very often do nothing to halt the progression of the curve. Really only effective in a skeletally immature patient, or as long as your child is growing, a brace does not improve the curvature, but if taken off for a long period of time, the curve has been shown to progress.

Many children who have scoliosis and wear a brace often participate in sports, including football. The danger then is not so much to themselves, but to their teammates or opponents, because the brace is very rigid and can injure someone in collision.

One of the most important factors in having a brace worn successfully in adolescence is participation of the family, especially in physically active pastimes. If this is not the case, very often the child resists the brace or does not follow exercise instructions.

Athletic performance at aerobic capacity does not change at all with a brace for curves under 50 degrees. As a rule of thumb, the endurance test in scoliosis youngsters suffers a 10 percent reduction with every 20-degree increase in curve. There is no change in aerobic performance when the curve just changes 5 to 10 degrees, so there is much room for excellent physical performance.

Scoliosis must not be taken lightly. A youngster with scoliosis needs the support of the family and should be counseled by a sports medicine physician or physiatrist. In later years, osteoarthritis may develop, and that can become a painful condition by imposing pressure on the nerve roots. When this happens surgical intervention may be required to relieve pressure on the nerve roots. But whatever the case, I cannot emphasize enough the importance of keeping the trunk muscles strong and limber.

SHIN SPLINTS

There are not too many popular songs about the time-honored science of anatomy, but I am told that virtually all American children grow up learning that "the shinbone's connected to the anklebone" from singing a wonderfully lively spiritual in school.

Well, the shinbone, or tibia, *is* connected to the anklebone, and it can become painful with overuse. Tibial pains are commonly called shin splints—supposedly an old Anglo-Saxon expression. Shin splints are caused by little tears in the tissue that attaches the anterior tibial muscle to bone. This muscle runs from the front of the foot up the front of the lower leg and on to its ultimate anchorage on the outside of the shinbone, or tibia. When you flex your ankle, as when you stand on your heels, the muscle tightens and provides power. If you overdo this in jogging, running, or jumping up and down (and remember, your feet land some 2,000 times in running a mile with an impact two and a half to three times your body weight), the muscle can become inflamed where it connects with the shinbone. It may even tear. The result: varying degrees of pain at a point halfway between your knee and ankle, most often on the outer edge of the bone and extending up and down for four to six inches.

This is the most common variety of shin splints. Another comes from having flattened arches and running a lot, in which case the problem may occur sooner and be more painful. For either variety, the treatment is the same: Stop jogging or running or training, and rest for at least a week. Ice applied every other hour while awake, for twenty minutes or so, and aspirin, will usually help the pain and inflammation, but the rest period is most important.

Shin splints should not be taken lightly, for the condition can mask two other problems, both of which may be highly painful and require careful diagnoses.

The first of these has the dramatic name of anterior compartment syndrome, and it, too, involves overexertion. Your lower leg is divided vertically into chambers, or compartments, that are surrounded by a tough material called fascia. The anterior compartment lies along the outer side of the shinbone and encloses three muscles, of which the anterior tibial muscle is one. When these muscles are overstressed they can become inflamed, a process that involves leaking of fluid from blood vessels into the compartment. Unfortunately, the fascia doesn't have much give, so as the swelling increases, so does the pressure within the compartment. This can restrict the normal flow of blood to the muscles, causing pain and even interfering with the functioning of the peroneal nerve, which makes the anterior tibial muscle work. This pain, which can be severe, will appear just to the outside of the shinbone, and the muscle weakness will be evident when you try to flex your foot. Ice and aspirin should help, but rest is most beneficial of all. Stay away from jogging or running for at least two weeks, then return gradually at half speed, giving the muscles in your anterior compartment time to adjust to the increased activity in your legs. In extreme cases, simple surgery may be necessary to

relieve the pressure, but I have never known of a case of anterior compartment syndrome caused by overuse that required surgical intervention.

I recently treated an unusual case of anterior compartment syndrome. A lovely young woman who wore high boots when she walked to work often took a short cut through Central Park, and one day, inspired by the beautiful scenery and the runners and bikers all around her, she started jogging. She kept up the routine, and to her dismay noticed that her ankle was getting weaker and weaker, day by day. The pressure from the top of the tight boot over the anterior compartment muscles served to increase the pressure within the compartment. The cure was relatively easy to figure out—stop running with tight boots on!—but it took the young lady several months to regain the strength of her ankle, given its weakened condition from damage to the nerve.

Instruments are now available to measure the pressure in the anterior compartment. Many sports medicine centers have them, though I seriously doubt whether being tested by them is really better than a good clinical examination, or whether it affects the ultimate outcome. I know of several patients whose anterior compartment syndrome improved, but whose pressure measurements didn't!

The second problem that shin pain may mask involves the shinbone itself. Overexertion again is the culprit, but this time it is the bone that absorbs the punishment and, like metal subjected to continued bending or pounding, finally cracks. This is called a stress fracture, and its description and treatment come under a separate section.

There are two exercises you can do after the acute stage of shin splints subsides. Both are designed to strengthen the anterior tibial muscle along the shinbone by making it work against weight. You should try to do these exercises twice a day. Remember to breathe regularly while exercising, and to relax completely between repetitions.

EXERCISE 1

This exercise will loosen and strengthen the anterior tibial muscles. Sit in a straight-backed chair with a rolled towel or sand-filled stocking placed under the thigh of your injured leg. Strap a 1-pound weight across the top of your foot (as close to the toes as possible). Flex your foot straight up toward your shinbone and hold for 5 seconds (count to 6), then relax for 2 seconds (count to 3). Start off doing 8 repetitions, and when you can do 12 easily, increase the weight by one pound, drop down to 8 repetitions, and begin building up to 12 again. Do this until you reach a maximum of 12 repetitions with 8 pounds.

EXERCISE 2

This uses the same starting position and weight as in the preceding exercise. Turn the foot out and up, and hold for 5 seconds (count to 6). Then return to the starting position and relax for 3 seconds (count to 4). This exercise loosens and strengthens the everter muscles, a pair that run up the outside of the lower leg. Start off with a 1-pound weight doing 8 repetitions, and build up to 12. When you can do 12 repetitions easily, increase the weight by one pound, drop down to 8 repetitions, and begin building up to 12 repetitions with a total of 8 pounds.

EXERCISE 1

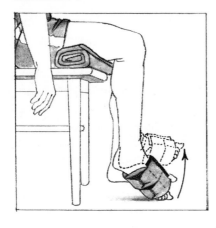

EXERCISE 2

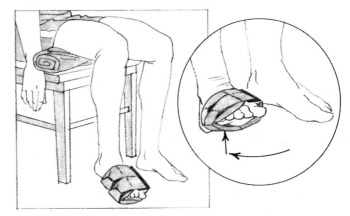

SLIPPED DISK

"Slipped" spinal disks, as they are known popularly, are a problem we see frequently at New York Hospital, though actual slippage is not involved at all. What happens is that the tough fibrous material that encircles the disk's jellylike center (the nucleus pulposus) suffers tiny tears and gradually loses its capacity to hold the soft core in place. The result: a bulge in the disk covering, one that may eventually press on a nerve root as it emerges from the vertebrae. If the disk covering actually ruptures, some of the soft inner material may ooze out and also press on the nerve. This is known as a herniated (ruptured) disk. Medical science is not sure exactly why these things happen in some people and not others, but it is clear that when any part of a disk presses on a nerve root, the person can experience excruciating pain, pain that will appear suddenly, shoot down one arm or leg, and increase dramatically, depending on one's movements and the position of the body. If, for example, you have a disk problem and I ask you to raise your leg with your knee straight while you are lying down, the pain may become especially severe in the leg. If the disk problem is in the neck, you will have severe pain in your arm when you tilt your head backward.

There are two ways to approach the problem of slipped disks: the conservative nonsurgical approach, and surgery. Treating you conservatively, we may put you to bed for a few days and give the disk a chance to dry out and shrink, and the surrounding inflammation to settle down. Then we would start you on a carefully designed exercise program to achieve a biomechanical advantage that will prevent further irritation and, one hopes, further episodes. However, this is not always sufficient. In about two out of ten cases that we see at New York Hospital, we have to call in a neurosurgeon to operate and trim away the troublesome portion of the disk. This is a major procedure, called a lami-

nectomy, because the surgeon removes the portion of the bony vertebral body called the lamina in order to get at the disk. After the surgery, we get you up right away and send you into the therapeutic pool, sutures and all, to keep your muscles from tightening up. The following day you would begin an exercise program for the lower back, and after a week, if all is well, you'd be sent home.

There are other types of disk surgery, but they should be considered very carefully. Microsurgery may be performed under certain circumstances, usually depending on the location of the damaged disk. It is done under a microscope magnification with very small instruments. The advantages of this technique are that it leaves a smaller scar and may permit the patient to leave the hospital sooner than would be the case with a laminectomy. The risk is that because the surgical opening—or the visual exposure—is small, a tiny disk fragment not in the visual field may be missed, and this could cause major post-surgical difficulties.

There is also a form of chemical surgery, pioneered in Canada, that uses an enzyme substance called chymopapain (it comes from the papaya fruit) to dissolve the nucleus pulposus inside a damaged disk covering. This procedure is not as simple as it sounds, however, and must be done under general anesthesia. In my opinion, it should be considered very cautiously. Injecting chymopapain into the disk may be an intriguing idea, but given all the patients I have seen whose chymopapain procedures didn't work out too well, I do not feel that the clinical results have justified all the fanfare. True, some people may leave the hospital after a day or two, but very often they have to visit a rehabilitation doctor for several weeks of physical therapy to relieve the continuing muscle spasm. I just don't believe that the long-term results of chymopapain intervention will substantiate the early enthusiastic reports of success, and I suspect it will gradually disappear from the medical scene.

Fusion is a procedure in which disks are removed and adjacent vertebrae are encouraged to fuse together after being packed with chips from the pelvic bone. Fusions were once done much more frequently than they are now, often in conjunction with a laminectomy.

While there is no such thing as a truly "slipped" disk, it is possible to have some slippage of one vertebra over another. This simple condition has the complicated name of spondylolisthesis. If the slippage is severe enough to cause severe radiating pain and instability of the spine, a fusion may be needed to remedy the situation. This is the most common indication for fusion nowadays, but I can recall only three or four such operations in the last fifteen years at New York Hospital. Unfortunately, we still see fusion patients for whom less heroic measures might well have been more effective. They come to us many years later with evidence of osteoarthritis that has developed in the vertebrae and facet joints both above and below the area of fusion.

The surgical outcome of spinal fusion is never certain even in the best of surgical hands, and your fusion may not become solid and "take." If fusion is offered to you, whatever the underlying cause of your back problem, you should obtain a second opinion to find out what other approaches are available to you. If the slippage is not severe, it can often be contained with a very diligent program of strengthening the stomach muscles.

Repeated back surgeries do not, in my opinion, improve the chances of relief. Of course, there are exceptions, times when there is no alternative course of action, but I think it fair to say that while one back operation often helps, two or three do so only rarely.

The decision whether or not to operate on a back problem cannot be made purely on the basis of radiologic studies or laboratory tests, unless there is evidence of a tumor in or around the spine or a disk fragment is jammed against the nerve root. If a piece of disk breaks off and jams into the area where the root emerges from the spinal canal, there is no way to dislodge it except by surgery. The pain the patient experiences is much worse than one would expect from the actual size of the fragment. We have no definite explanation for this, but there may be some irritative chemical reaction between the nerve root and the fragment.

The most important factor by far remains the clinical picture. Not all radiating pain in the legs is caused by a bulging or herniated disk. Trigger points and muscle spasms have to be excluded with certainty. Many patients who have evidence of damage to the nerve—such as diminished or absent reflexes in the leg; a positive straight leg raising test, which aggravates the pain; or even weakness in the leg—do very well with a carefully structured and monitored nonsurgical program. People with disk problems should really be given a chance to see how they can do without surgery, and not be rushed into anything. I always prefer to monitor such patients, together with a neurosurgeon or neurologist who can help detect subtle changes in the clinical picture.

We recently did a follow-up study at New York Hospital on 700 back patients with lumbar disk disease, patients who had had X-rays, CAT scans, myelograms, and electrodiagnostic tests. We found that there was *no* direct correlation between the degree of abnormality shown on these tests and the patients' response to surgical or nonsurgical treatment.

In the rare cases where a loose fragment is diagnosed on a CAT scan, or a nucleus pulposus is completely herniated (something that occurs very rarely), neurosurgical intervention is usually required. In most instances, however, the nonsurgical approach to a "slipped" disk is preferable to the surgical approach.

Lack of interest in the non-surgical treatment of low back problems by the medical profession has brought many self-appointed specialists into the field: chiropractors, muscle therapists, etc. Some of them developed certain theories, many of which have not been confirmed. One such theory is to push the disk back into place by doing extension (or "back-arching") exercises. There is absolutely no evidence that this will happen though the exercises may help to relax back muscles and, as was mentioned, muscle relaxation is one of the main therapeutic targets to aim for in acute backs. And if the muscles can be loosened up with extension exercises, they should be done. But any other therapeutic claim has not been substantiated. Extensive studies have shown that eventually it is the strengthening of the abdominal muscles and of the back extensor muscles as well as the stretching of these muscles that eases the pain of a slipped disk.

SORE KNEE

There are a number of terms that honor the complexity of the knee joint. One that sounds appropriate without actually telling you anything is "internal derangement of the knee." Indeed, if your knee hurts, it is highly probable that something between the femur and the tibia may be "deranged," or out of place. But then comes the question, what? And this is the only question that counts. Another term is "extensor mechanism insufficiency," which is a fancy way of suggesting simply that you have a weak quadriceps—that four-part muscle (the body's most powerful conglomerate) that fills your thigh and provides the knee with much of its operational stability. A good way to manage this problem is to strengthen your quadriceps.

"Chondromalacia of the patella" is another case in point. Though this term turns up regularly on insurance forms, it means little more than having a sore knee. The pain is caused by a roughening and irritation of the cartilage of the kneecap, changes that do not normally show up on X-rays.

Chondromalacia of the patella can develop with any activity that requires knee action. Eighty-five percent of the time the problem can be handled without any major diagnostic studies or surgical intervention. If chondromalacia of the knee is the likely diagnosis, there should be both a short-term approach and a long-term approach for handling it. The short-term approach is geared toward pain relief, usually achieved by decreasing or stopping athletic activities for three to four weeks. The long-term approach is to do whatever you can to prevent a recurrence. One such measure is to strengthen the knee extensor muscles. If your pain were very severe, especially when you walked, I would advise you to use crutches and keep your weight off the painful knee during the strengthening period.

In most instances, your quadriceps would already have weakened because of your favoring the affected side, so you should start on strengthening exercises fairly soon. These should be "reduced arc" exercises that put less stress on the patella and its cartilage than the usual 90-degree flexion-and-extension type of exercises. The knee is bent to 30 degrees and then has to come to full extension with weights around the ankle. The weight resistance schedule should be adhered to as outlined in the exercise instructions. One can also do just straight resistance training—that is, exercise with weights—for the quadriceps with the knee in complete extension. The weights should be increased very gradually. Once you reach five to ten pounds, the exercises need no longer be done daily; three days a week would be sufficient. For continuing athletic activities, one can use a patellar brace, or a so-called chondromalacia strap, that is applied right beneath the kneecap and helps its gliding motion.

It is also important to be evaluated for malpositioned feet, which may have contributed to the problem. If this is the case, you should have custom-made orthotic devices for your shoes to help prevent further problems. Arthroscopy or any other invasive study should be reserved only for very severe cases that don't improve.

SPORTS MEDICINE

With the recent increase in athletic pursuits by an ever higher percentage of the population, including people in middle age, a field of sports medicine has emerged. This is not, however, a formal medical specialty requiring specific training and board examinations. Any physician or hospital can establish a sports medicine clinic.

The physicians most likely to be involved in treating sports-related injuries are physiatrists, orthopedic surgeons, and family practitioners. Ninety percent of such injuries can be taken care of with proper physical therapy techniques and exercise, and, if necessary, protective and orthotic devices such as splints and braces. Only about 10 percent require surgical intervention. (People sometimes ask why we don't put up a "Sports Medicine" sign in our department, and I explain that we have always treated musculoskeletal injuries democratically! We are happy to treat a rotator cuff tear whether it comes from playing football or from yanking a suitcase off an airport carousel.)

Most people who participate in athletic activities and regular exercises have a genuine desire to return to them as quickly as possible. They are generally, by their nature, activity-oriented, disciplined, and geared toward improved performance.

This makes them good patients, and this quality along with their need and desire for sound medical advice and guidance has already generated a great deal of useful clinical experience and research data. Physicians who take care of a lot of sports injuries are becoming more and more knowledgeable about them and about the specific needs of individual situations.

Childhood injuries require special attention because they may adversely affect the growth of bone, with potentially devastating effects in adulthood. I would recommend seeking the advice of a pediatric orthopedic surgeon, a pediatrician, or a physiatrist in such situations.

As far as surgical intervention is concerned, I believe this should, in most cases, be reserved for the professional athlete, or anyone else whose livelihood depends on the quickest possible return of function. The average patient—for instance, with a rotator cuff tear—can do very well with a structured rehabilitation program and no surgery. It will just take a little longer.

Some sports medicine clinics perform cardiac evaluations, including stress tests, and design aerobic programs for cardiovascular fitness. It's fine to engage in such programs, but if you are over thirty-five, I think it's a good idea to have a cardiologist analyze your condition.

There is still much to be learned, and the jury is still out as far as the merits of certain approaches to sports injuries are concerned. For example, a five-year follow-up study on anterior crucial ligament injuries in the knee has shown that the results of surgical and nonsurgical approaches are about the same. More studies of this kind need to be done, but for now I believe the best thing sports medicine can do for a patient is to take all factors into consideration and formulate a tailored, individualized approach.

SPRAINED ANKLE

The ankle, separate from the bones in the foot, is one of the more vulnerable joints of the body. It has a structure that moves basically in two directions, upward (dorsiflexion) and downward (plantar flexion). Ankles take quite a beating day in and day out as they carry our weight around and absorb a pounding with each step, and if we don't use them properly they incur problems. Certainly they are not very well constructed to tolerate tripping or turning under, and sprained ankle is one of the most common of all injuries. With all-too-painful frequency it happens to the young (though generally not before the teens) and the old, the athletic and unathletic.

You can sprain your ankle doing almost anything, from stepping off the curb to tripping on a rock or falling over someone else's foot. In addition, you may have a tendency to walk on the outside of your foot (supination), which will more than likely turn your ankle inward and subject it to a sprain. And if you've suffered a number of sprains, you may have permanently loosened the outer ligaments in your ankle, which will make you still more vulnerable to turning it.

What happens when you sprain your ankle? The most common sequence, called an inversion sprain, is that your foot suddenly turns in under you, you momentarily lose balance, and the weight of your body slams down hard on the bones and ligaments in the joint. This stretches not only the ligaments but also the joint capsule, a tough, fibrous material that encloses the joint. Small blood vessels rupture, fluids flood the area, and the ankle swells and becomes painful. This is the simplest of ankle injuries with ligaments, bone, and capsule essentially intact. It is known as a Grade I sprain.

What should you do when you sprain your ankle? If you are outdoors, you should get home quickly, putting as little weight as possible on the injured ankle. If you can, take a taxi or have someone drive you, or call someone to come and pick you up. Don't be fooled by the absence of pain in your ankle: For the first half hour or so, your ankle won't seem so badly off, and pain and swelling will be minimal. I assure you that it will get worse!

It's important to be aware that there are three kinds of ankle sprains because each requires a specific treatment approach. If, after forty-eight hours, you put weight on your ankle and it still hurts, you may have a Grade II sprain and should see a doctor. Most family physicians have had a great deal of experience treating sprained ankles and will know how to grade them. You can help by answering your doctor's questions as specifically as possible and not hiding any pain or discomfort. If it is a Grade II sprain, a cast should be put on for at least four to six weeks so that the joint is immobilized and the torn ligaments have a chance to heal. This may seem a long time to have your ankle in a chunk of plaster,

and I am perhaps conservative in my treatment, but I feel that it is considerably better to endure temporary discomfort than to hobble on a painful ankle for the rest of your life. If you choose not to wear a cast, then at least use crutches for those four to six weeks.

In such a situation, your physician probably will take an X-ray of your ankle to rule out a fracture of one of the malleoli, certain bones on the side of the ankle. If a malleolus is indeed fractured, you will have to wear a cast for six to eight weeks.

If you sprain your ankle at home, begin the following treatment at once. Stay off it and keep it elevated—that is, keep your leg up on a chair or some pillows. During the first twenty-four-hour period apply an ice bag or cold pack for twenty minutes every hour while you are awake. At the end of this period, if there is little or no pain, try walking on the foot. If the ankle is still swollen and continues to throb, use crutches if you have to get around and continue icing for another day. If you have suffered a Grade I sprain, this should be the end of it.

It can be difficult to distinguish between a Grade I and Grade II sprain, and the distinction is important. In a Grade II sprain you may have actually torn portions of the ligaments that hold your ankle bones together. If this is the case, and your ankle is not treated properly, then the sprain will heal but the joint may become loose and slip from side to side as you walk. If this continues, the cartilage that pads the bones in the joint will erode, and once *this* happens there is no way to reverse the process. Your ankle will hurt you chronically and you may require surgery, or at the very least some form of orthotic support. I have had so many patients tell me: "Ever since I had that fall, my ankle has been hurting me." When I hear these words, I can't help but wish that a proper diagnosis had been made at the start.

While Grade II sprains are somewhat difficult to diagnose, Grade III injuries present no diagnostic problem at all. For in addition to considerable pain and swelling, a Grade III sprain involves actual separation of the ligament or ligaments. This can occur in two ways. First, the ligament may tear apart. In this case, an orthopedic surgeon will have to stitch it together. Some physicians may do a stress X-ray, which means they will X-ray your ankle in an extremely turned-in position to see indirectly whether there is a complete separation. The ligaments won't show up on the X-ray, but the position of the ankle bones will give a clue. (Most physicians can tell the difference between Grade I, II, and III ankle sprains just by examination.)

The other type of Grade III sprain occurs when a small chunk of the bone that anchors the ligament is pulled off with the ligament still in one piece. This is called an avulsion injury, and if an X-ray confirms it a cast must be put on so that the bony chunk and ligament will reattach to the bone. It is possible that a Grade III tear will heal without help, but you can't count on it. You and your orthopedic surgeon will have to take action: sew it up and put a cast on. I've heard too many older people say, "Every time I step down, my ankle turns over." This is probably from a Grade III sprain that was not treated properly, and the ligaments never grew back together.

The exercises that follow can help in three ways: to strengthen the muscles that control ankle motion, so that you will be less likely to suffer sprain; to reduce the stiffness of the joint capsule; and to rebuild muscle strength after a sprain. Care should be taken to ensure that the motion of the "hind foot" is restored to normal after a sprain, or else your ankle will be vulnerable to future sprains. The exercises should be done twice a day. Remember to breathe regularly while exercising, and to relax between repetitions.

EXERCISE 1

This exercise is designed to strengthen your ankle. Sit in a straight-backed chair and place a rolled-up towel under your injured leg and a 1-pound weight on the instep of that foot (*not* around the toe). Flex your foot toward your shin, being careful not to move the rest of your leg. Hold this position for 5 seconds (count to 6), then lower and relax for 3 seconds (count to 4). Work up to 12 repetitions, then increase the weight by a pound and start with 8 repetitions again; work up to a total 8 repetitions with 6 pounds.

EXERCISE 1

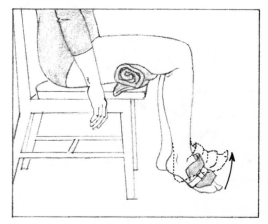

EXERCISE 2

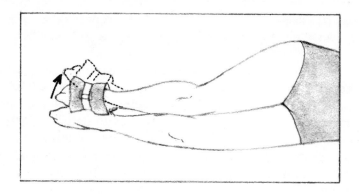

EXERCISE 2

This exercise is designed to strengthen the muscles on the outside of your lower leg, the peroneal muscles. Lie on your side with your injured ankle on top and a 1-pound weight on the outside of your injured foot, just below the ankle bone. Flex your foot to the side without bending your leg. Hold for 5 seconds (count to 6), then relax for 3 seconds (count to 4). The rest period between repetitions is important: It gives your muscles a chance to recover. Start off with 8 repetitions and work up to 12. When you can do 12 repetitions easily, add a pound, drop back to 8 repetitions, and work up to 12 again. Continue until you reach a total of 12 repetitions with 6 pounds. More than 12 repetitions will not increase strength and it may tire the muscle. Lying down while doing this exercise reduces the swelling of the ankle.

EXERCISE 3

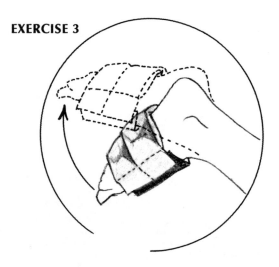

EXERCISE 3

This exercise is designed to strengthen your calf muscle (the most important in the lower leg) so that it will not atrophy while your ankle recovers. Lie on your stomach with a pillow under your abdomen and a 1- or 2-pound weight strapped to your toes. Bend your knee and lift the lower leg to a

45-degree angle; try to point your toes up toward the ceiling. Hold this position for 5 seconds (count to 6), then drop your toes (but not your leg) and relax for 3 seconds (count to 4). When you can do 12 repetitions easily, add a pound and drop down to 8 repetitions. Your goal is to do 12 repetitions with 3 or 4 pounds.

STIFF NECK

The medical term for stiff neck is acute torticollis. This may sound impressive, but what it refers to in ninety-nine out of a hundred cases is nothing more than an extremely common and painful crick—a pain in the neck, or a stiff neck. You can get it in any number of ways. For example, you may play tennis or squash, which will heat you up and make you perspire, then afterward you may stay around to chat or have a cooling drink; if you cool down too quickly, or a little breeze blows on your neck, this may be enough for the long muscles on the side of the neck (the paracervicals) to go into spasm. The same thing can happen when you suddenly move after you have held one position for a long time and have overstretched the muscle, or the muscle may be too tight—that is, not relaxed enough for the motion you intend.

The most effective treatment is to put ice on the area for fifteen minutes, then do exercises to slowly loosen the tightened muscles. And you can take Tylenol or aspirin for a day or two to dull the pain. You can even have your neck X-rayed, but the X-rays won't show the muscle spasm directly, and they won't change the course of treatment; they will show only a straightening of the natural curve in the neck that results from the tightening up of the muscles.

A stiff neck is mainly a problem of muscular spasm. One treatment I would strongly advise against is to put your neck in a traction device that would apply either a steady or intermittent pull on the muscles over a period of several minutes. Because the mechanical force of the muscle in contraction—that is, in spasm—is much greater than the mechanical force that can be applied with such traction, the only result will be more pain. You are putting stress on a muscle that is already in spasm, and most likely the spasm and pain will get worse. In order for traction to be effective, the muscles have to be relaxed. This relaxation is best achieved with the application of ice packs and, sometimes, gentle electrical stimulation to the right muscles. The physiatrist or physical therapist who first sees you may spray the painful muscles with ethyl chloride, which is very cold and will dull some of the pain, before putting you through some loosening exercises.

Three exercises that will help loosen the muscles that support your head and neck are described on page 249. Do them slowly and carefully, and be sure to breathe regularly as you work. Don't hold your breath, and relax completely between repetitions. If the pain and stiffness do not start to subside in thirty-six hours, you should see a physiatrist or orthopedic surgeon.

Just remember, the idea is to *ease* your muscles out of their spasm, not wrench them out of it. If you try to overpower your tightened muscles, they will probably overpower you with pain.

EXERCISE 1

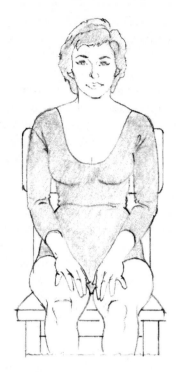
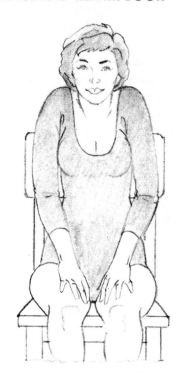

EXERCISE 2

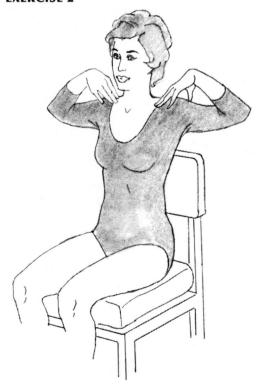
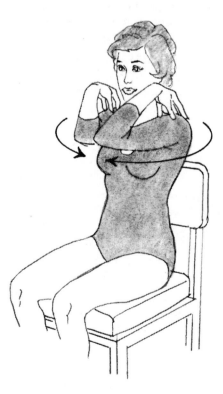

EXERCISE 1

Sit in a straight-backed chair with your feet flat on the floor. With your hands resting in your lap, slowly raise your shoulders toward your ears as far as you can without straining. This upward movement should take about 5 seconds (and may hurt slightly). Then let your shoulders slowly return to the normal position. Relax to a count of 3 between each repetition, and concentrate on keeping your fingers and shoulders as loose as possible. Do 5 repetitions once every hour following ice treatment.

EXERCISE 2

This exercise helps to loosen the trapezius muscle, often the culprit in stiff necks. Raise your elbows to shoulder height, place your fingers on your shoulders, spread your elbows back as far as you can, then bring them together in front of you. Hold this position for 5 seconds (count to 6). You should feel a gentle pull in your upper back and neck. Relax by dropping your hands into your lap. Do 5 repetitions once an hour along with ice treatments and the first exercise.

EXERCISE 3

This exercise is designed to loosen the posterior neck muscles. Sit or stand as relaxed as possible, slowly turn your head to the right as far as you can, then slowly turn it back to the midline. Rest 1 or 2 seconds. Repeat to the left. The turning from midline to the side should consume about 5 seconds (count to 6). When you return to the midline, rest again for 1 to 2 seconds. Repeat this exercise 5 times.

EXERCISE 3

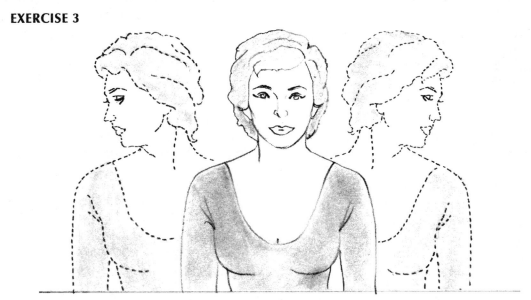

STOMACH MUSCLES

If you could do only one exercise, what should it be? Probably the sit-up, an exercise that for years was taught in gym classes and military training camps with the legs straight out. We have since learned that this is not an optimal position because it makes the hip flexors contract and takes away some of the work that the stomach (really abdominal) muscles should be doing. It also puts more pressure on the lower back and gives you a higher chance of hurting it, especially if you are older. Doing sit-ups with the knees bent is more effective because it makes your stomach muscles work harder.

The sit-up is as basic to good posture and proper body alignment as the muscles it strengthens. These are the abdominals, a remarkable package of four layers of overlapping, crisscrossing fibers: the rectus abdominis, strongest and closest to the surface, which runs from the ribs down to the pelvis; the internal and external obliques, which weave diagonally from opposite sides; and the transversalis abdominis muscles, which extend from side to side and, essentially, from front to back across the abdominal cavity.

What makes the abdominals so important? In this instance the obvious is also the significant: The stomach muscles occupy a central position in the body, lying in a kind of muscular transition zone between torso and legs, and if they are firm, their effect will be beneficial on the total alignment of the body. Strong abdominals will eliminate unnecessary stress on the muscles in the back, and even in the upper legs. They constitute one muscle group that you definitely do not want to stretch. Loose abdominals can contribute to muscle strain and spasm in the lower back, for they won't provide adequate balance for the back muscles, and they won't hold internal organs firmly against the spine. They can, on the other hand, create a condition known as hyperlordosis, or swayback, in which the low back arch deepens and this posture can be responsible for triggering painful muscle spasms.

Do not depend on stomach muscle exercises to decrease the circumference of your waistline. This can only be done by losing weight! You can, however, succeed in flattening your abdomen by doing daily abdominal strengthening exercises.

What's the best way to do sit-ups? Below I've listed five ways to perform the exercise in increasing order of difficulty. The basic correct way to do any sit-up is to "roll" your body up. If you suddenly jerk up, you will have momentum doing most of the work and your abdominal muscles will not get the benefit. Lift your head off the floor first, then your shoulders. You thereby roll up to prevent straining your neck. To roll back to the starting position, reverse the sequence so that your head touches the floor last. You must remember to inhale before you start the exercise, exhale through pursed lips as you sit up, and breathe in again after you come down.

As with any exercise, start with the easiest version to lessen any risk of injury. And remember that pain and strain do not add to the value of any exercise. All it is likely to do is leave you stiff and sore, and decrease your chances of continuing with your exercise program.

EXERCISE 1

This is perhaps the easiest way to exercise and tighten your abdominal muscles. Get down on your hands and knees—knees under hips, hands under shoulders. As you exhale, drop your head and draw your abdominal muscles up into your body and hold for 5 seconds (count to 6). Return to the starting position, then relax for 4 seconds (count to 5). It's especially important to take a deep breath at the start of the exercise, and to exhale while you draw in your stomach muscles. Begin the exercise with a small number of repetitions, say 3 to 5, and gradually work up to 10. After you can do 10 repetitions easily, you're ready to go on to the next level of difficulty.

EXERCISE 1

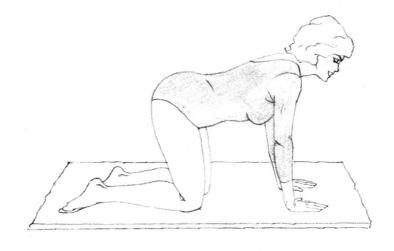

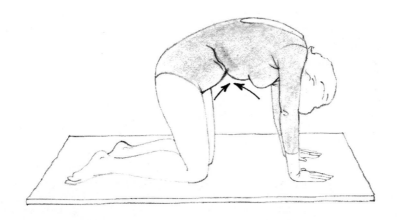

EXERCISE 2

Lie on your back with your arms at your sides, knees bent, and slightly apart, and feet flat on the floor. As you exhale, raise your head, upper back and arms as far off the floor as you can without straining. At first you should simply roll up gradually into a half sit-up position, then roll your body back to the floor, and breathe in.

Relax between repetitions. When you first begin doing this exercise, you may find it necessary to secure your feet in place under a couch or heavy chair. After a few days you may want to hold the up position for 5 seconds (count to 6) and then drop back and relax for 4 seconds (count to 5). Start with a few repetitions, then gradually increase to 15 repetitions, without straining.

EXERCISE 2

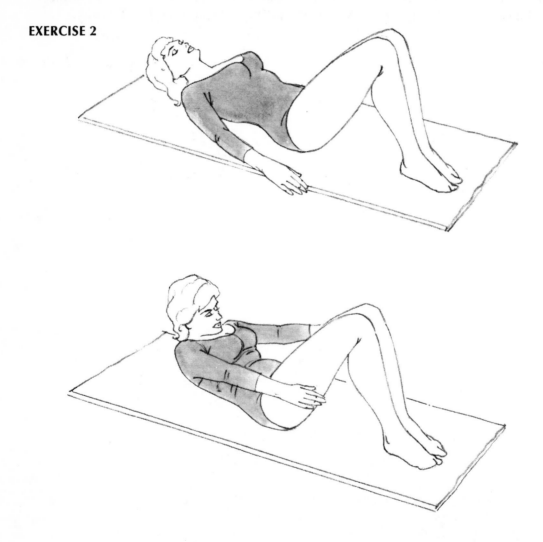

EXERCISE 3

This is done in the same position as the previous sit-up, but this time bring your arms up so that they extend beyond your knees and your forehead comes as close as possible to your kneecaps. Return to starting position and relax. When you first begin doing this exercise, you may find it necessary to secure your feet in place under a couch or heavy chair or have somebody hold down the feet. If you want to increase the effectiveness of the exercise, try to consume 5 seconds (count to 6) on the way up, and 5 seconds (count to 6) on the way down.

EXERCISE 3

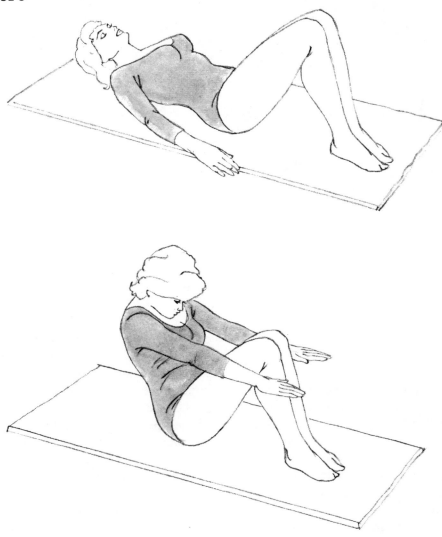

EXERCISE 4

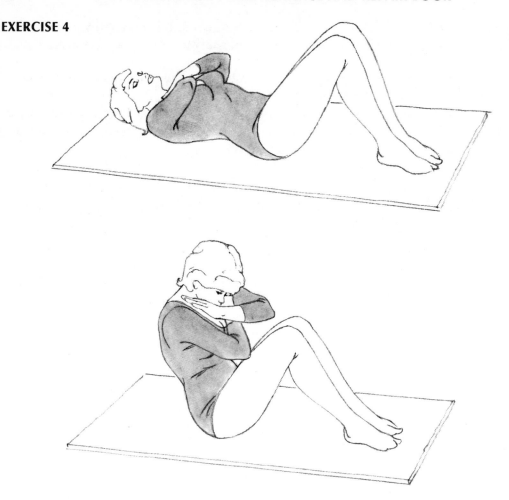

EXERCISE 4

There are a number of variations of the full sit-up. One involves doing the exercise with your hands across your chest. When you first begin doing this exercise, you may find it necessary to secure your feet in place under a couch or heavy chair. If you want to increase the degree of difficulty, clasp your hands behind your neck, or hold weights (2 or 3 pounds) behind your neck or around your upper arms. But, as with all sit-ups, you have to be very careful not to strain your neck. This is why it's always important to roll-up. Still another variation includes turning the trunk as you come up, first to the right for a number of repetitions and then to the left. If you can already do a dozen or so forward sit-ups, turning the trunk is a good idea; it helps strengthen diagonal abdominal fibers. Remember to relax between repetitions and to exhale as you sit up.

EXERCISE 5

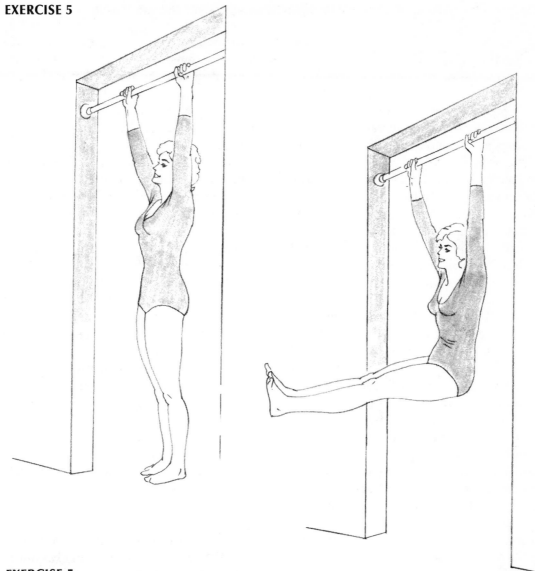

EXERCISE 5

This most difficult abdominal exercise of all is one of the simplest to explain. First, hang from a bar, legs fully extended. Then, bending your knees, draw your legs up to your chest and straighten them so they're parallel to the floor. To place an even greater demand on your abdominals, do the exercise as slowly as you can, raising your legs straight in slow-motion and lowering them in the same manner. Remember to exhale as you bring your legs up, and inhale as you lower them. The ultimate stomach muscle strengthener is to bring your straight legs as far up as possible. You have to have strong arms and strong abdominal muscles to do this.

STRAIN AND SPRAIN

These terms are often confused and misused, probably because they sound alike. Both do refer, however, to varying degrees of damage to complex soft-tissue systems.

The word *sprain* refers specifically to damage of ligaments, the tough, inelastic fibers that bind the bones in your joints together. An easy way to remember the meaning of the term is to think of one of the most common of injuries: a sprained ankle. The bony ankle joint is held together by four major ligaments, and thus when you sprain it, you injure one or more of these fibrous bands. Sprain damage is generally graded by category, there being three rankings in all. A Grade I sprain involves minor temporary damage to one or more ligaments, along with some irritation of the joint capsule and rupture of small blood vessels. There is, however, no interruption of the anatomical integrity of the ligament or joint capsule. Fluid simply leaks out from the injured blood vessels and causes swelling. In a Grade II sprain, the ligament may actually be frayed, the swelling and discomfort may be more extensive, and, most important, the joint may be unstable. Grade III sprains occur when a ligament is completely torn or ruptured (which frequently occurs when it is stretched more than 5 percent of its length), or when a chunk of the bone to which it is anchored breaks loose—an avulsion injury. Such injuries require careful diagnosis and immobilization of the joint in a cast. For more on sprained ankles, see page 243. A sprained wrist, often a less severe injury, also involves damage to the ligaments.

Strains, on the other hand, affect the tissues—the muscles and tendons—that supply and deliver the power that makes our joints work. Strains are also graded by degree of severity and occur in a variety of locations. Many involve partial ripping in the center, or belly, of a muscle, but the majority take place at the connection between muscle and tendon. A few involve actual tearing of tendon from bone. In a Grade I strain the fibers are overstretched rather than torn, and discomfort should not last longer than a few days. A Grade II strain is more serious, with numerous muscle fibers actually torn. This causes bleeding into the muscular tissue, which can then trigger a severe muscle spasm reaction. In a Grade III strain major damage has occurred—the muscle is essentially ruptured (though I personally have never seen a muscle completely separated from its tendon). Grade III injuries require immobilization and a long period of healing and rehabilitation, as much as four to six months depending on the size and location of the injured tissue. Sometimes the muscle will have to be sutured together by a surgeon. Regardless which is your own situation, you will need a very structured rehabilitation program under expert guidance. Otherwise you will be highly vulnerable to reinjury and unable to participate in many activities. Therapy will require a substantial amount of work on your part, but the effort is worthwhile.

STRESS FRACTURES

The development of a stress fracture is somewhat like metal fatigue: repeated stress to a bone causes tiny cracks in its structure (as opposed to the sudden, out-and-out type of break that you would get in a skiing accident, for instance). The area then becomes painful and vulnerable to further injury.

Before participation in athletic activities became so widespread, it was thought that stress fractures occurred only in the bones of the foot. Such fractures were initially observed in soldiers who had to march over long distances carrying heavy packs, and were thus called march fractures. But now, with the growth of organized sports and better record-keeping methods, we know that stress fractures can occur in nearly any bone that is subjected to cumulative stress by physical exertion. We see them especially in tibial (lower leg) bones of runners and in the pelvic bones of women athletes.

It can be difficult to diagnose a stress fracture because the symptoms may mimic a number of other conditions—pelvic stress fractures in women, for instance, may be mistaken for gynecological, abdominal, or hip problems. That is why it is important for the physician to pinpoint the time of pain onset and correlate it carefully with a history of the patient's activities. Also, a stress fracture often doesn't show up on an X-ray until several weeks after an injury, when evidence of natural bone healing processes to repair the area first become visible. It is sometimes necessary to order a bone scan, which is more sensitive than an X-ray in detecting stress fractures. This involves injecting radioisotopes into the bloodstream, which then accumulate around the area of any stress fracture and show up on the scan as a darkened spot.

A stress fracture will heal well in a few weeks if you cut down on, or eliminate, the activities that caused it. In the old days, plaster casts were used, but this is no longer necessary. If you are a runner or jogger, and your stress fracture is in the tibia, stop running, avoid standing on the leg for long periods or walking for long distances, and use a cane to take some of the weight off the affected leg. If you have been doing strengthening exercises for your legs using ankle weights, stop doing them. You can keep exercising in other ways to maintain your aerobic condition—swimming is good because it doesn't require your legs to bear any weight. After about six weeks from the onset of symptoms, new X-rays should be taken to check on signs of bone healing. If they are evident, you may start running again, but you should ease into your program gradually, allowing about eight to ten weeks to get back to your original condition.

Incidentally, running downhill and running on hard surfaces substantially increase your chances of incurring a stress fracture, and being on a crash diet with a low calcium intake also heightens the risk—two things to keep in mind if you're on a running program.

STROKE

Disruption of the flow of blood to any part of the body can have serious consequences. If heart-muscle cells are deprived, the result may be the nagging pain called angina. If the supply is blocked completely, cells will die and a heart attack will occur. If the supply of blood to the lower limbs is impeded because of a narrowing or stiffening of the blood vessels, the result may be pain, heightened sensitivity to cold, and, in extreme cases, complete blockage of blood flow and the onset of gangrene.

Four major blood vessels serve the brain—the body's command center—two arise on either side of the neck and two pass through openings, or foramina, in the vertebrae of the neck. All are vulnerable to blood-flow problems, as are the large and small blood vessels within the brain itself. Partial or complete blockage of any of these vessels can cause damage to the brain. Such cerebral injuries, which may be slight and transient or serious and life-threatening, are lumped under the term "stroke."

Though the death rate from stroke in this country has declined substantially over the last decade, about 400,000 Americans suffer new attacks each year, and 165,000 die as a result of strokes, making the disease a leading cause of death after coronary problems, cancer, and diabetes. Those who initially survive strokes offer a unique health challenge, for they require sensitive, painstaking rehabilitation and care for both physical and emotional problems.

What can cause such destructive disruptions in crucial cerebral blood vessels? Clots that form *within* the brain (thrombi) are one cause, with the cerebral incidents they precipitate preceded in some cases by a brief period of disorientation, slurred speech, numbness, dizziness, and disrupted vision. These symptoms constitute what are known as transient ischemic attacks, or TIAs, and it is important that you recognize and report such episodes to your doctor. Immediate treatment can delay or eliminate more serious problems later on. Cerebral blood vessels may also rupture (hemorrhage), squirting blood into brain

tissues and damaging or killing vital cells. And then there is an embolism, or clot, that has broken off and traveled from another site (such as the heart) *into* the brain, where clogging of the blood vessel occurs, as in the case of thrombi.

Risk factors for stroke include hypertension (high blood pressure), smoking, overweight, genetic tendencies, and diabetes.

For whatever reason and however it may occur, damage to the cells that sense and direct human operations inevitably affects mental and physical function, sometimes in slight, barely recognizable ways, and in other instances with profound disabilities, impaired mental function, and loss of speech. As a result, if you or anyone in your family suffers any of the symptoms mentioned above, however briefly, your first step should be a quick, direct trip to your doctor and, if he or she feels it's necessary, immediately on to a hospital or medical center experienced in the assessment and treatment of strokes and in stroke rehabilitation.

The first few days following a stroke are crucial, both in terms of medicating and treating the patient and in assessing the kind and degree of damage that has occurred. Neurologists have special skill in taking care of a stroke in its acute stage. The rehabilitation process will start very soon after that.

The most common type of stroke involves thrombosis of the middle cerebral artery and produces the disabilities most often associated with a stroke: partial paralysis on one side (because of the brain's crossover wiring system, the side opposite the damaged cerebral hemisphere), with the arm more affected than the leg, and with loss of control of one side of the mouth and, occasionally, the tongue. Because the upper portion of the face has nerve representation in both brain halves, while the lower segment does not, brain cell damage on one side will often knock out the function of the lower face on the opposite side.

Other kinds of damage may also occur, and it is important to know and remember them. Strokes can damage the swallowing reflex, for example. They can also affect the victim's sense of spatial orientation, and even reduce his field of vision. Visual field defects are a little tricky to detect but can cause great difficulty for the patient. A neurologist should monitor them along with other changes in the neurologic exam as rehabilitation proceeds.

Brain cells that die because of insufficient oxygen cannot regenerate. The same holds true when heart muscle cells die in a coronary occlusion. Should you suffer a stroke, however, it is most important to realize that structured rehabilitation exercises—that is, specific programs tailored to your disability—can retrain new muscles to perform lost functions. Such relearned motions won't be as smooth as those you have lost (after all, it took you years to learn them in the first place), but you can develop them through careful, repetitive movements, just as you did as a child. So, a certain degree of repatterning is possible and can produce remarkable results, if you are prepared to do the work required. What is crucial, however, is that the disabilities created by your stroke be assessed, expertly and completely, and that the exercises you are given be specifically designed to improve those disabilities, or at least

compensate for them. It is also essential that you learn to do your exercises correctly, under the guidance of the physiatrist who directs the rehabilitation team working with you.

Perhaps most important in stroke rehabilitation is the mental state of the patient and those around him or her. For an independent, physically active person, the sudden stroke-induced loss of function is invariably devastating. The helplessness that results can be overwhelming, and the need to depend on others for even the simplest of tasks, like putting on clothes, seems humiliating. Eventually, it is important for the physician to sit down and discuss everything very specifically and realistically with the patient and the patient's family: what has been achieved; what can be achieved; and what, in all probability, it may not be possible to achieve. If a person has outside interests such as walking or gardening or hiking, then with hard work he or she should be able to continue in a way and to a degree that is satisfying. But if the patient has been a competitive recreational athlete and finds he can no longer compete, then he may not accept compromise and will be unwilling to stick with an exercise program. The usual result: He may sit around and become depressed.

If you are severely disabled after a stroke, you may need to spend some time at a rehabilitation center with special programs for stroke patients. Physical and occupational therapists will work with you intensively on exercises, on walking, and, in general, on learning how to become as independent as possible in daily activities. Sometimes splints and other assistive devices will be made or provided for you. A speech therapist will work with you, if necessary. And family members should be shown how to help.

The thing to remember is this: If you don't give up and keep working, you can accomplish a *great* deal.

TENNIS ELBOW

Some years ago I was visited by a remarkable patient, an eighty-one-year-old gentleman who was extremely fit and played tennis with the drive and tenacity of a much younger man. When this vigorous octogenarian told me that he was suffering sharp pain on the outside of his elbow, I could hardly believe it. Surely his playing habits had been well-established by now, and certainly his body, despite his age, was sound. When I asked him what had happened, he told me the following: He had been losing, perhaps not surprisingly, to younger players and had decided to make some changes. He had altered his grip, changed his racquet, and switched from his old-fashioned underhanded serve to a more modern and dynamic overhead smash. Shortly thereafter the pain in his elbow had appeared, and had grown worse until he finally called me and made an appointment. He had indeed developed tennis elbow. Why? Because he had made a number of alterations in his game, some seemingly minor, some major, and the muscles in his forearm were not prepared to meet the challenge.

The man's story points up the essence of the tennis elbow problem: change and inadequate forearm firepower. But first let me clarify the term "tennis elbow," for it is,

so to speak, a "double-faulted" term—both misleading and inaccurate. Though there are more than 35 million regular tennis players in this country, and almost half can expect to experience the misery and frustration of tennis elbow, millions of people who don't play tennis will suffer from it as well. They may be mechanics or bowlers or gardeners, or even eager politicians who have shaken too many hands. And so the term is misleading. It is also inaccurate because sufferers don't have pain inside their elbow; they feel it on the outside of the joint just above the elbow crease. Pain appears here because it is the point at which the major muscles in the forearm are anchored to the upper-arm bone by a tendon, the point where irritation and roughening can occur if forearm muscles are asked to do more than they are used to. Two motions are especially responsible for delivering punishment to the tendon: repeated tight gripping while turning the palm upward (supination) or tight gripping while turning the palm downward (pronation). These are the motions employed in driving a screw into hardwood no less than in whacking a forehand with more enthusiasm than technique.

If you were to arrive at my office with a sore elbow, whether you are eighty-one years old or thirty-one, I would listen to you very carefully, because your story would indeed be a crucial element in forming my preliminary diagnosis. At first you may say that the pain started a few days ago or just last week, but then, on reflection, you may add that it hurt just a little six weeks ago, or even longer, and that the elbow has been getting worse ever since. If the pain has developed gradually, then you are probably a member of the largest club of tennis elbow sufferers. Officially, you have a problem at the lateral "epicondyle." This is where the tendon of the wrist extensor muscles, the muscles that move your wrist back, attaches to the upper bone of your elbow joint. And this is why tennis elbow is technically known as *lateral epicondylitis.* Interestingly, the problem rarely appears before the age of fourteen, when the lateral epicondyle, the bony prominence the tendon is anchored to, becomes fully developed. The stressful and repetitive gripping and turning you have been doing have translated into irritation, even roughening on the underside of the tendon where it glides over the bone. Seventy to 80 percent of tennis elbow sufferers share this same problem. Nor does the structure of the affected tendon help much. Unlike most of your tendons, this one has neither a protective sheath nor lubricating fluid to bathe it, so it is prone to irritation.

Having reached this conclusion, I can test my diagnosis in a number of ways. I can ask you to hold your wrist back while I press down on it, or to hold an object tightly, or to turn your forearm against my resistance—all with your elbow straight out. If the elbow is bent or flexed, the tendon does not have to glide over the irritated area, and you will not feel any pain. If, on the other hand, the pain gets worse and is localized just above your elbow, I can be reasonably certain that the tendon is the culprit. I will then examine your arm even more carefully in order to pinpoint the location of the irritation. Is it where tendon and muscle meet? Is it in the space between the tendon and the bone it is anchored to? If you have already had many

bouts of tennis elbow, you may have developed a bursa right under the extensor tendon known as Osgood's bursa. This is the body's protective reaction against repetitive iritation, but unfortunately it too can become painful.

When I have learned as much as I can, and if the pain and irritation appear to be moderate, I may suggest that you use ice and aspirin to reduce your discomfort. But if the tissue beneath the tendon is extremely irritated, I will probably give you an anti-inflammatory injection. I will carefully locate the very tender area over the lateral epicondyle, and then mark the skin. You will barely feel my injection because I freeze this area first with a surface anesthetic (ethyl chloride spray). This not only spares you some discomfort, it also keeps you from jumping when my needle punctures the skin! No question, it helps my markmanship considerably.

The next day, for about twenty minutes, I will apply mild electrical stimulation (pulses designed to mimic normal muscle contractions) to the muscles that move your wrist (wrist extensors). Gradually, those muscles will begin to loosen up. In two or three days the acute pain should be relieved, and you will be ready to begin the crucial process of rehabilitation that is absolutely essential if you wish to avoid further aggravation at your lateral epicondyle—that is, a recurrence of tennis elbow.

There is always the possibility that you aren't suffering from either of the conditions I have described but are a member of a more exclusive branch of the tennis elbow club. You may have essentially the same kind of pain that most other sufferers have, but it will be on the *inside* of your arm, at the *medial* epicondyle, where a second major tendon anchors another sheath of muscle to bone, this time the wrist flexor muscles, which bend the wrist downward. For every seven cases of lateral epicondyle irritation, we turn up one such "inside job." The wrist flexor muscles that insert on the medial epicondyle become actively stressed from a strong overhead serve or at the end of the golf swing when there is sudden flexion of the wrist. That's why medial epicondylitis is also known as golfer's elbow. In contrast to the backhand, where the wrist extensor muscles are the most stressed and do most of the work, serving overhead in tennis and swinging through in golf stress the flexor muscles most. Initial treatment for this condition is the same as that for the more common variety.

Maybe you belong to *still* another group of sufferers. Your original story about the sudden onset of pain may be similar, and a specific, recent incident may have triggered your discomfort, but your problem will be at the musculo-tendinous junction where muscle joins to tendon, rather than where tendon meets bone. This means that an impact to your arm, perhaps delivered by a whizzing 50 mile-per-hour volley or a 90-mile-per-hour serve—or through some other means, such as hammering vigorously or chopping wood with a hand axe—has torn some of the muscle fibers that join the tendon. After my diagnosis I may have a splint made for your wrist, set back at about a 30-degree angle, so that your wrist extensor muscles will be as relaxed as possible. After that I'll apply electrical stimulation to these muscles. I will not inject any medication, but I may use ethyl chloride

spray to help reduce the pain. In two or three days the acute phase should be over, and it will be time for you to start exercising.

Believe it or not, there is still *another* problem for tennis players, called tennis *arm*. Here the pain is really in the muscles of the forearm rather than at their attachment points at the elbow, or at the muscle-tendon junction. The condition may be seen in enthusiastic gardeners who overdo their spading and shoveling in the planting season. Basically, it results from overusing and straining two sets of muscles in the forearm: the supinators (which rotate the forearm) and the wrist extensors (which move the wrist back). When abused, these muscles become swollen and painful. If you tighten your grip and rotate your forearm, the pain will start at your wrist and run rapidly up your arm. The condition appears most often after a vigorous first session of tennis (or squash or paddle tennis or gardening) after months of inactivity. In the days before indoor courts and winter tennis, this meant a dramatic rise in the number of cases of tennis arm in early spring. Now such seasonal peaks are less prevalent.

Proper treatment of these tender forearm muscles includes a splint to immobilize the wrist, the application of ice, and exercises designed to strengthen the forearm once it has had a chance to rest. It is important to give this common muscle problem sufficient time to heal. If you don't, the injury may bother you the entire season, and it even may increase your chances of developing tennis *elbow*. How long should you wait? In most cases until all signs of pain have subsided, including when you test the muscles against weights. Then, if you do play again and experience pain the next day, you should stop altogether, reassess the situation, and consider seeing a physiatrist.

There are some instances—I will cite two—in which surgery may be your best, and possibly last, avenue of treatment. If, after about a year, conventional exercise techniques (to be described at the end of this section) have failed to help your irritated and possibly frayed tendon, you may want to consider surgery. The operation is a relatively simple procedure, one designed to lengthen the roughened tendon and thus reduce its tendency to scrape over bone. About five out of a hundred tennis elbow sufferers ultimately decide to undergo such surgery. Other patients, after suffering through various painful episodes over many years, may develop so much swelling at the muscle-tendon connection that the thickening will press on the branch of the radial nerve that runs down the forearm. The result is nearly constant pain, and surgery is invariably necessary.

In the vast majority of cases, however, surgery is not required. The acute pain should go away in two or three days. It is really not as difficult as you imagine at the time. But only you, the person who is actually gripping and turning that screwdriver or straining to whack that backhand or forehand can know exactly what is going on and where the overload is coming from.

Fortunately, considerable research has been directed at this problem, since it affects millions of people. Studies with pressure gauges placed inside racquet handles have shown that expert players (who rarely develop tennis elbow) hold their racquets loosely before impact, then tighten as they swing. The amateur or weekend player, however, is likely to grip his racquet tightly all the time, placing heavy, unrelieved pressure on the forearm muscles. And then there is poor backhand technique, which can affect your elbow as much as your game. The player who relies on the twist of his elbow and wrist to power his backhand, instead of using his body and shoulder, is most likely to suffer (players with a two-handed backhand rarely do). Not hitting balls on the sweet spot of the racquet stresses the forearm muscles more to absorb the torque. Excessive rotation on forehand drives, and net play with the arm out of position rather than poised at a 70-degree angle (considered optimal for absorbing the force of impact) can also deliver damaging stresses to the forearm and elbow. Self-analysis is the first and most important phase of your treatment, so I suggest you sit down and think your way back to the episode of physical excess or the sequence of twists and turns that triggered your attack. This may not have been clear in your mind when you first saw your doctor, but if it then becomes clear you should discuss it with him and see what adjustments you could make without causing further injury. It also might be wise to take some lessons with an experienced coach.

Our studies have shown that weak forearm muscles increase your chances for tennis elbow. You may benefit from one or more of the following exercises. They are what we recommend to patients with tennis elbow at The New York Hospital–Cornell Medical Center.

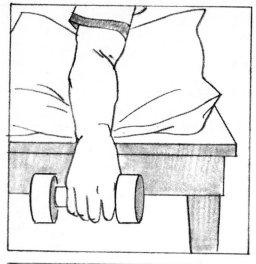

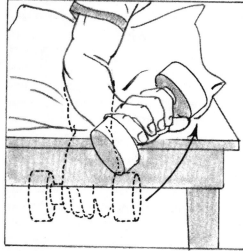

EXERCISE 1

This exercise strengthens your wrist extensor and, even more, the extensor carpi radialis. Firmly grip a 2- to 3-pound weight with your playing arm. Place your forearm, palm down, on a solid surface of books or hard cushions—your wrist should be positioned at the edge of the support—so that the hand gripping the weight hangs free. Bend your wrist upward and toward your thumb, so that your thumb points to your body, and hold for 5 seconds (count to 6). Return to starting position and relax for 2 seconds (count to 3). Repeat 10 times; gradually work up to 12. When this gets easy, add a pound, go back to 8 repetitions, and work up to 12 repetitions with 10 pounds.

EXERCISE 2

This exercise strengthens your wrist flexors. Grip a 2- to 3-pound weight with your playing arm. Place your arm, palms up, on a pile of books or hard cushions—here, too, your wrist should be positioned at the edge of the support. Bend your wrist

EXERCISE 1

EXERCISE 2

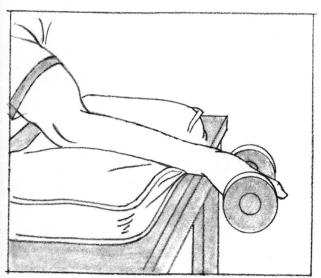

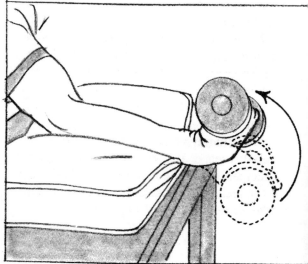

upward toward the ceiling as far as you can and hold for 5 seconds (count to 6). Return to the starting position and relax for 3 seconds (count to 4). Repeat 8 times and gradually increase to 12. When you can do 12 repetitions easily, add a pound, go back to 8, and work up to 12 repetitions with 10 pounds.

EXERCISE 3

This exercise strengthens your forearm rotators. Grip a 2- to 3-pound weight with your playing arm. Place your forearm, palm down, on a pile of books or hard cushions; your elbow should be bent. Slowly rotate the forearm clockwise 180 degrees, turning your palm upward. The movement should take 5 seconds (count to 6). Return to starting position and relax for 2 seconds (count to 3). Repeat 8 times and gradually increase repetitions to 12. When you can do 12 repetitions easily, add a pound, go back to 8, and work up to 12 repetitions with a total of 10 pounds.

EXERCISE 4

This exercise is designed to train your fast-acting muscle fibers (the ones that are needed for sudden movements) and follows the movement in the preceding exercise. Begin with a 3-pound weight, or half the weight you ended up using in the above exercises; do 3 sets of 8 repetitions *quickly* with *no rest period* between repetitions and no more than a 1-minute rest between sets. When you can do 3 sets of 12 with a 3-pound weight, add a pound and go back to 8 repetitions per set, then work up to your goal: 3 sets of 12 with 6 to 8 pounds. Do not increase weight or repetitions at any level if you feel pain or strain either during or after the exercises.

EXERCISES 3 and 4

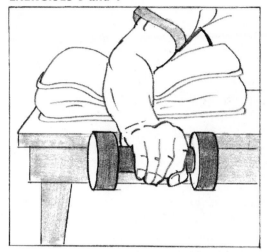

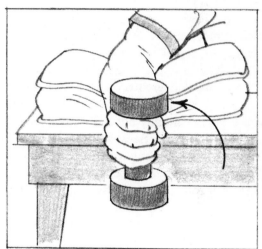

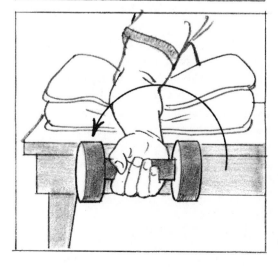

TENS (TRANSCUTANEOUS ELECTRICAL NERVE STIMULATORS)

These are small, battery-powered devices, about the size of a transistor radio, that work effectively on many patients to reduce or block pain signals before they reach the brain. Developed in the 1970s and viewed with skepticism for a time, these stimulators are now accepted and widely used with success.

The TENS battery pack is wired with two or more electrodes that you the patient attach to specific locations assigned by your physician. Tiny amounts of electrical current are delivered through your skin to the nerve fibers beneath it, overloading those neural circuits normally involved in transmitting pain. Because of the natural limits of the loading capacities of such fibers, the technique blocks out or restricts signals before they reach your brain. The pack may also help your body release endorphins, natural painkillers found in the brain, but much more research needs to be done before a more definite explanation can be given.

Patients generally use TENS signals intermittently, switching the current on for half an hour to an hour at a time. Many report a slight vibration or tingling sensation when the device is on. The system may be used to treat any type of pain that does not warrant medical or surgical intervention. I must point out, though, that many patients do *not* respond to TENS, in the same way that they may not respond to certain medications. Still, it is worth trying. I usually prescribe TENS for patients who are in too much pain to undergo a physical therapy program and who, in my opinion, could be taking less medication for pain control. One of the system's principal virtues, in addition to easing pain, is that it reduces the need for painkilling medication without added risks. This is important because as we get older almost all of us end up taking some medication for something. Thus, any pain-relieving treatment that works by using simple physical means can be valuable to one's general well-being.

TRACTION

In certain specially selected cases of pain radiating from the neck to the shoulder, upper arm, and forearm, traction can accomplish a great deal by adding a tiny bit of distance, about one millimeter (the thickness of a dime), to the overall span of the four lower vertebrae in the neck and cervical spine. Such cases involve pain caused by what is known as nerve root pressure, or a pinched nerve. Although it may seem a modest goal, one millimeter of breathing room may be just enough to ease the pressure on the nerve and give a patient two or three years of relief.

What causes the pain? Pairs of nerves emerge from each side of the spinal cord passing through openings (foramina) in the vertebrae to various parts of the body. Osteoarthritic changes can narrow and roughen these openings, putting pressure on a nerve root and causing intense pain. Or the fibrous covering on a disk may tear and eventually rupture, releasing the soft material inside that then presses on a nerve and produces the same sort of pain. When this happens, either because of bone changes or disk pressure, the result is known as *cervical radiculopathy*. It can happen to anyone, but most frequently the problem appears in people in their late forties and fifties as bones and disks undergo the changes of aging.

Do radiating pains in your neck and shoulder make you a candidate for traction? In many cases, yes, but not always. If you were to come to me with neck and shoulder pain, for example, there are a number of conditions I would have to eliminate before I decided that you might benefit from traction. Could you be suffering from spinal cord damage or compression? Could your pain be referred pain coming from another site, such as your heart or gallbladder? Could muscle spasms or trigger points be the cause of your misery?

Laboratory and radiologic tests are not always helpful, and they can even confuse the picture at times. I remember one patient, a young man who had been told that he was suffering from nerve root compression because of certain abnormalities that had turned up on his CAT scan. After high doses of oral steroids had failed to help him, surgery was suggested. He had come to me for a second opinion. When I examined him, I found muscle spasm and trigger points in his neck. After a few weeks of physical therapy for these problems, he was free of pain. His tests had shown abnormalities, but they had not been the cause of his discomfort.

If bony protrusions or a disk are indeed pressing on a cervical nerve, and traction might be helpful, one should proceed the way I suggested above. We carefully check for and eliminate any muscle spasms or trigger points we may find. Why "carefully"? Because if neck muscles are in spasm and we were to try traction right away, the contracting force of the spasm would be greater than the pull of traction. As a result, the procedure would fail, and the traction would only add to the pain already in the neck.

After we've zeroed in on the diagnosis and eliminated muscle spasms, the time to begin traction in the hospital under professional guidance will be at hand. In my opinion, home traction devices are not very effective. Though I firmly believe in self-help when possible, I don't believe that cervical home traction falls into this category. Not that such devices are useless, it's just that in my experience they don't provide the same therapeutic benefits as an electrically controlled, intermittent cervical traction device applied and monitored by a skilled physical therapist.

Intermittent cervical traction is a safe therapeutic device. I don't know of any serious complications. If the pain seems to be aggravated by the traction, then it is probably because muscle spasm and trigger points were overlooked during the first examination and have to be taken care of.

The only time I wouldn't use traction for a cervical radiculopathy is if you've had surgical fusion in your neck. Traction would be useless and probably risky.

If you come to me as a candidate for cervical traction, I first explain what is going to happen. You start the treatment by sitting in a comfortable chair, head tipped forward at about 40 degrees—the angle is important (and hard to establish and maintain at home on your own) because in this position your foramina are opened to the fullest. Your head is supported by a padded chin strap with attachments front and back. These are hooked to the device that holds the weights that apply pressure to your neck. The pull is delivered intermittently at regular intervals, not steadily, because this is how people can best tolerate it.

Once you are comfortably settled, we start at 10 pounds of pressure, then move up to 15 or 20 pounds. Our goal is to deliver about 35 pounds of pull to those four crucial vertebrae in your cervical spine. To do this we may actually have to put 50 or so pounds on the machine, but it will take a number of sessions before we reach this point. Usually, each session will take about fifteen or twenty minutes. You may require a dozen or so to obtain relief from radiating pain and the benefits may last for several years before you have to undergo traction again. In addition, the second time you come for traction you will probably need fewer sessions.

People often ask me about wearing cervical collars when they have a pinched nerve in the neck. While these offer no true mechanical support, they can be helpful for a couple of weeks in limiting the motion of the neck and preventing further irritation of the nerve. Sometimes it helps to wear them at night to avoid positioning the neck in a disadvantageous way.

It is also possible to operate on the cervical spine to relieve nerve pressure. Many surgeons are reluctant to do this, however, except in those cases where there is no alternative, because the upper back and neck constitute such a complicated nerve center.

The lumbar, or lower, spine is not amenable to traction. It would take at least 600 pounds to stretch your lower spine, and this couldn't be done without causing tremendous pain.

The vertebrae of the spine are held tightly together with very strong ligaments, muscles, and joint capsules. In the neck region you can stretch the neck muscles and joint capsules, with intermittent cervical traction, just enough to cause a slightly forward-angled separation between the vertebrae that make it easier for the nerve to pass through the opening alongside. In the lower back, however, the muscles are much larger and more powerful and cannot be stretched to a significant enough degree. So if you see someone with low back problems in traction in a hospital bed, you will know that the traction is really doing little more than making sure the patient stays in bed. Notes in the chart like "Today the patient was able to tolerate 10 to 12 pounds of traction" are not true indicators of the patient's progress when related to the lower, or lumbar, spine.

TRIGGER POINTS

Though more and more doctors are detecting and treating these hard, painful knots in muscle tissue, trigger points remain something of a mystery to the public and, for that matter, to large segments of the medical community. They shouldn't, for they are common, relatively easy to locate, and can be removed with the proper technique.

Trigger points are hard, tangled lumps of muscle fibers that probably started as muscle spasms and then, because they were not released, turned into painful nodules. Biopsies have shown trigger points to be composed of degenerated muscle tissue. Such pain-producing knots are usually located in the center, or belly, of a muscle. In the hip and shoulder region especially, trigger points can mimic the symptoms of nerve root pressure, and if detected and properly treated they and the pain they cause can be eliminated, and the patient can be saved from an expensive work-up for spinal pathology (and possible misdiagnosis).

In 1931, a German orthopedic surgeon, Dr. Hans Lange, wrote a major work on the subject of trigger points, and in the 1960s Dr. Hans Kraus, a well-known physiatrist, treated President John F. Kennedy for trigger points in his back. Trigger point injections, combined with physical therapy, are among the tools that can be useful in overcoming back and neck problems.

How do I detect the presence of trigger points? Though they often appear in the neck and shoulders, they can also plague muscle groups in the legs and lower back. The procedure I follow is slow and painstaking: I move the tips of the fingers of my right hand slowly over the area that seems to be affected, pressing lightly on the back of my right hand with the fingers of my left. When I find a trigger point, I move my fingers slowly back and forth across that area until I am sure of its location. Then, even when I press gently on the knot, the patient will feel it, and may wince or jump or even cry out with pain.

In certain cases it may be possible to break up trigger points with heavy massage or electrical stimulation, but in most instances it is necessary to inject them with a mixture of local anesthetic and saline solution. The anesthetic helps mask the sting of the needle as I penetrate the perimeter of the trigger point, and the saline solution, which has the same osmotic, or membrane-passing, pressure as tissue fluid, forces the clumped-up fibers apart. This is a mechanical, not a pharmacological treatment.

Once the nodule has been broken up, rehabilitation of the muscles in the area can begin. This consists of electrical stimulation to the involved muscles in order to make them contract and relax more rhythmically again. The stimulation is tolerated well by the muscles and is not painful. Treatments should be followed by gentle limbering exercises, and after two or three days stretching and strengthening exercises should be added. In my experience, trigger point injections without the proper follow-up treatments are of no value. The pain will usually recur.

Trigger point injections are just one auxiliary measure in a total rehabilitation program, although usually a very important and effective one. The risk involved when they are given by a competent physician is minimal. I do not, however, recommend doing more than one or two trigger points at one time; otherwise one can confuse the whole picture of the pain pattern.

Many variations of trigger point injection have been recommended recently. One is dry needling, in which a fine acupuncture needle is inserted into the trigger point and no fluid is injected. This is followed by stretching exercises right after needling. There is no evidence that this technique is superior to the trigger point injection program described above, although investigations are going on, and it is possible that sometime in the near future we may modify our basic approach to trigger points accordingly.

ULTRASOUND

Ultrasound is a very useful modality in physical medicine and rehabilitation because it allows heat to be generated more deeply into the body tissues than does any other form of treatment. Hot packs and heating pads are by definition superficial forms of heat, and such deep-heating methods as short-wave and microwave diathermy, while they do send electromagnetic waves through the tissues, do not send them as far as ultrasound, and are more difficult to aim and adjust accurately.

Ultrasound waves are generated by electrically induced vibrations from a crystal, but they themselves are *mechanical,* not electromagnetic, waves. They are similar to those employed in fetal scans of pregnant women, though they operate at a different frequency. When ultrasound waves strike tissue, the tissue vibrates and heats up. In joints, the waves bounce off bony surfaces and become even more effective at generating heat. Used when there is no longer any acute swelling, ultrasound can be aimed effectively and is most often employed in the localized treatment of tendinitis, bursitis, and especially bursitis of the hip. The waves will travel right through fatty tissue and muscle to the joint, where they hit bone and are converted to heat. Muscle tissue is also heated up, but only by about one-tenth as much as bone.

Along with improving blood flow, sound wave vibrations block the formation of adhesions in injured tissue. Patients often expect ultrasound treatments to involve a machine so gigantic as to make the body shudder from its bombardment of sound waves, but nothing could be further from the truth! An instrument the size of a microphone is applied to your skin and gently moved back and forth with a "coupling" cream used to help conduct the sound waves through the skin. You may feel some warmth in the area that is being treated, but that is all.

Sometimes ultrasound is used with a special cortisone cream, and then it is called phonopheresis. It is thought that the ultrasound waves actually drive the cortisone deeper into the tissue to provide an additional anti-inflammatory effect, but the ultimate proof for this has not yet been established. Still, its clinical usefulness is quite well-accepted, for in rehabilitation, as in other fields of medicine, the principle of usefulness is applied even if a detailed mechanism of action has not been fully elucidated. The same holds true for many beneficial pharmacological agents.

Ultrasound treatments are given in series

and must be carefully monitored to ensure that excessive and potentially damaging heat is not produced. Ultrasound should not be used near the eyes, the reproductive organs, the liver, or over areas of numbness and poor blood supply.

WEATHER AND HEALTH

There is no question that changes in barometric pressure and movements of weather fronts have an influence on health. I don't know of anyone who isn't sensitive to weather changes one way or another. Even people who believe that they're absolutely insensitive to weather are in fact sensitive! The cells and fluids in our bodies have to expand and contract according to the laws of nature. As far as the musculoskeletal system is concerned, we might feel the effects of such fluctuation as pain in a joint, or a headache, or general muscular fatigue. It is a well-established fact that arthritis sufferers are weather-sensitive. They often know ahead of time what the weather will be, and I must say their predictions are nearly as accurate as those of professional weather forecasters! People who have suffered an injury will also feel a resurgence of pain when the weather changes. Anyone who has undergone surgical fixation of a fracture—attachment with screws, bolts, or rods—will feel these weather changes, too, because artificial or man-made inserts have a different "accommodation gradient" than living bone. Even very healthy children are often quite sensitive to increases in temperatures: Their systems are not yet sufficiently developed to be as impervious to heat input from the outside as is true of adult systems. On the other hand, there is no doubt that a healthy adult body also has the capacity to adjust to many changes in temperature and humidity, and is much less likely to feel the effects of weather changes.

It is important to understand that weather changes can cause an increase in, or a recurrence of, symptoms in your musculoskeletal system, even if you haven't increased your activities or done anything to hurt yourself. Otherwise you may worry unnecessarily over such symptoms.

How should you approach a weather-related aggravation of symptoms? Some people say "Ignore it and keep on going anyway—work through the pain!" To some measure I think this is a good idea. However, I've never seen weather-related pain get better by *increasing* one's activities; on the contrary, it gets worse.

Increased pain or discomfort as a result of weather changes, especially in the joints, can discourage people from exercising, even make them stop altogether for a while, but in most cases I think this would be wrong. No harm will be done if you continue, though if you don't feel quite up to your usual routine I would recommend cutting back a little and decreasing your level of activity. As with so many other things in life, exercise can and often should be adjusted to the climate. Weather-related pain will usually go away in one or two days, and then you can resume your regular level of activity. Nothing is lost in the way of physical fitness in such a short period of time, if you cut back a little.

WHIPLASH INJURY

This injury is commonly associated with automobile accidents, but it also occurs on the football and soccer fields, and occasionally the basketball court. It results from a powerful blow delivered directly to a person, or to a vehicle carrying the person, either from the front or rear. The impact of the collision takes advantage of the upper, or cervical, spine's most important capacity: flexibility. The head snaps forward or back, depending on the direction of the blow, then in whiplike fashion cracks back on itself again.

The damage may be slight, moderate, or quite severe, and it may involve straining or tearing the muscles that support the neck and spraining the ligaments that bind the seven cervical vertebrae to each other. Whiplash can also affect the nerve roots that pass out through the holes in the vertebrae (foramina). These openings are narrowed when the neck is thrown back, and the nerves, for a fraction of a second, are compressed and become irritated. Whiplash injuries can be more painful when you're older because after fifty these openings are already narrowed by the process of osteoarthritis; the sudden drastic pressure on the nerves passing through may be much greater than in a younger person.

Pain of whiplash may be severe at first and then abate only to return the next morning. Adding to the pain is the likelihood that your muscles will go into spasm, forming a kind of natural protective splint to immobilize the injured structures. Such spasms can be extremely painful and make treatment more difficult and complicated.

X-rays are of little help in determining the extent of damage to soft tissues, and the only change that will show up in cases of whiplash will be a slight flattening of the curve normally found in the back of your neck, caused by the pull of muscles that are tight and in spasm.

If I were to see you as a whiplash patient, I'd first check and make sure that you hadn't suffered any serious nerve damage. Then I would gently move your head and neck, trying to pinpoint the extent of muscle and ligament damage. Finally, I'd send you home with orders to use ice (every three or four hours) and to do the exercises at the end of this section to ease your pain and loosen your injured muscles. In two or three days, I'd have you come back for another exam and some electrical stimulation to relax your muscles. I'd also advise you to continue doing the exercises, twice a day at least, to keep your muscles from tightening up. And I might suggest that you buy a soft cervical collar. Though such devices don't provide true mechanical support, they do remind you not to move your neck any more than is necessary. And if you have to ride to work on a crowded subway, it will keep people from bumping into you! I would recommend that you wear such a cervical collar not longer than two weeks, then, for the next six weeks or so, wear it only when you ride in a car, or on a long plane trip, or when you have to sit for a long time at your desk.

The important thing to remember about whiplash injuries is that they can cause a great deal of discomfort and may last a long time. You should go to a physiatrist or neurologist right away and make sure that between the two of you the damage is treated and repaired with care and thoroughness. The main goals in the treatment of whiplash injury are to keep the muscles very loose while they are still painful, and then, since they will become weak from relative immobilization, undergo a strengthening program.

The exercises that follow will help loosen neck muscles injured by whiplash. They should be done at least twice a day. Work gradually and in consultation with your doctor; your neck muscles are very sensitive to stretching, and if you overstretch them you will only create more muscle spasms and pain. It is also important to relax and eliminate all tension in the neck muscles between repetitions. And remember to breathe regularly while doing the exercises.

EXERCISE 1

Sit in a straight-backed chair with your feet flat on the floor and your hands resting in your lap. Slowly raise your shoulders toward your ears, as far as you can without straining. This movement should take about 5 seconds (count to 6) and may hurt a bit. Slowly drop your shoulders to their normal position. Be sure to relax properly (count slowly to 5) between each repetition, and concentrate on keeping your fingers and shoulders as loose as possible. Do 5 repetitions.

EXERCISE 1

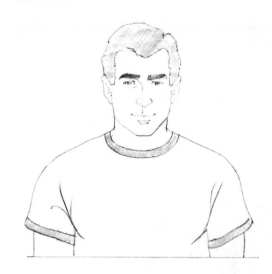

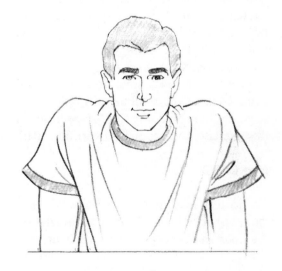

EXERCISE 2

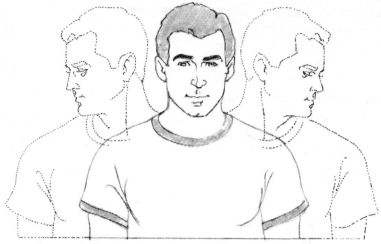

EXERCISE 2

After two or three days you can begin to stretch your neck by gently turning your head from side to side. Slowly turn to one side, do not hold, come back to the mid-line, and relax for 2 seconds (count to 3). Repeat to the other side, don't hold, and come back to the midline and relax for 2 seconds. Start off doing 4 to 5 repetitions of this exercise and gradually work up to 10.

EXERCISE 3

To do this neck flexion exercise, sit in a straight-backed chair with your feet flat on the floor and arms hanging loosely at your sides. Start with your head level and re-laxed, then slowly bring your chin toward your chest, stopping when you feel pain. Hold this position and breathe slowly until you feel the pain and tension ease. Then try to bring your chin down a little farther and repeat the breathing routine until the pain and tension ease. Continue bringing your chin toward your chest in this manner

until you reach your final pain tolerance level. Hold this final position for 5 seconds (count to 6), then slowly raise your chin to the starting position and relax for 2 seconds (count to 3). Start off doing 3 repetitions and gradually work up to 6.

As a variation of this exercise, after you

EXERCISE 3

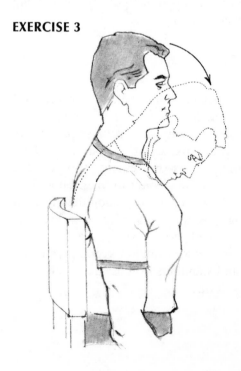

have brought your chin toward your chest as far as possible without straining and have reached your final pain tolerance level, try to slowly turn your chin toward one shoulder and hold for 5 seconds (count to 6). Bring your chin to the midline and relax for 2 seconds (count to 3), then bring it toward the opposite shoulder and hold for 5 seconds (count to 6). Finally, bring your chin back to the midline, slowly lift it up to the starting position, and relax completely. Start off doing 3 repetitions and gradually work up to 6.

Index

ABOUT THE AUTHORS

WILLIBALD NAGLER, M.D., born in Austria, received his medical education at the University of Vienna and trained at both the Hospital for Special Surgery and The New York Hospital–Cornell University Medical Center. Among other appointments and honors, he is Professor of Rehabilitation Medicine at Cornell University Medical College, Anne and Jerome Fisher Physiatrist-in-Chief at The New York Hospital–Cornell University Medical Center, and Chief of the Rehabilitation Service at Memorial Sloan-Kettering Cancer Center. He is also a member of the Advisory Board for Rehabilitation Medicine at The Hospital for Special Surgery in New York. His patients have included the late President John F. Kennedy, as well as many famous musicians, sports figures, and business leaders.

Irene von Estorff, M.D., born in New York City, received her liberal arts degree from Wellesley College and her medical degree from the Mayo Medical School, in Rochester, Minnesota. She is Assistant Attending Physiatrist at The New York Hospital, Clinical Assistant Physiatrist at Memorial Sloan-Kettering Cancer Center, and Assistant Professor of Rehabilitation Medicine at Cornell University Medical College.